Rapid Review

Medicine in Old Age

Dr Michael Vassallo
MD, FRCP(Lond), FRCP(Edin), DGM(Lond), M.P⸱ ⸱hD
Consultant Physician in General Internal Medicine a⸱⸱ ⸱ ⸱Medicine
The Royal Bournemouth Hospital, B⸱ ⸱ ⸱
and
Honorary Senior Clinical Lecturer, ⸱ ⸱ JK

Professor Steph⸱ ⸱⸱len
BSc, MBChB, MD(Manc), FRCP(Lond), FRCP(Edin), MBA
Consultant Physician in General Internal Medicine and Geriatric Medicine
The Royal Bournemouth Hospital, Bournemouth, UK
Visiting Professor of Clinical Gerontology, Bournemouth University, Poole, UK
and
Honorary Senior Clinical Lecturer, University of Southampton, UK

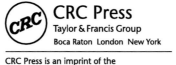

CRC Press
Taylor & Francis Group
Boca Raton London New York

CRC Press is an imprint of the
Taylor & Francis Group, an **informa** business

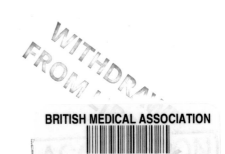

Disclaimer

Medical knowledge and best practice are constantly evolving as new research and experience contribute to our understanding. While the authors have taken every effort to eliminate inaccuracies, readers are advised to consult the most current information available on procedures, products, dosages, and formulae. Drug licensing varies between countries; the information given in this book mainly reflects UK practice. Neither the Publisher nor the Authors assume any liability for any injury and/or damage to persons or property arising out of or related to any use of the material contained in this book.

Acknowledgements

The authors wish to thank the following for permission to reproduce photographs: Michael Richardson (Figure **57**), University of Utah John Moran Eye Centre (Figure **26**), Lithuanian Society of Gerontology and Geriatrics (Figure **16**), and National CJD Surveillance Unit (Figure **22b**).

Preface

This book has two main purposes; formative case analysis and self-assessment of medicine in old age. It presents clinicians with a series of clinical cases that form the basis for discussion of the investigation and management of the patients. It also provides the trainee, or established doctor, with a medium to help prepare for post-graduate examinations and clinical practice. We believe it will be particularly useful to candidates taking the MRCP Part 2 written examination, the DGM, and formal knowledge tests for specialist registrars in Geriatric Medicine, General Medicine and Acute Medicine.

We have not attempted to write a comprehensive textbook of geriatric medicine as the field is vast and overlaps with many other specialties. Instead, we have chosen cases that cover the main modes of presentation of acute illness in old age, such as falls, confusion, incontinence, weight loss and immobility, with examples from all the major systems. These illustrate the complexity of diagnosis and treatment of medical illness in frail older people, and the need to think widely and laterally when caring for such patients.

All the cases are based on real people who have been under the care of the authors, and almost all the photographs are from the original patients.

The questions are mostly in best-of-five format, to reflect the current style of multiple choice questions used in examination, though we have included some open questions when that is more appropriate for the topic and as a basis for the tutorial sections. We have expanded many of the clinical stems to a size that is rather larger than that encountered in examinations. This provides a platform for a sequence of questions in the longer cases that improves the educational function of the book and more rigorously tests the reader's deductive thinking. We have phrased some questions in the negative. This reflects the reality of decision making in clinical practice, so we believe it is justified. Some topics and themes appear more than once; again, this is deliberate and serves to reinforce certain important messages.

We have used the past tense for all the clinical stems, though we have made free with the present and past tenses in the follow up sections according to the need for clarity, emphasis and a natural style. We hope the past tense purists among the readership will forgive us for taking that liberty.

Michael Vassallo
Stephen Allen

Classification of Cases

Note: references are to case numbers and not page numbers.

Cardiovascular disease 14, 33, 43, 53, 54, 55, 66, 88, 99, 101

Cerebrovascular disease 2, 13, 30, 44, 45, 109

Dementia and psychiatric disorders 5, 8, 22, 29, 59, 84, 95

Dermatology 4, 21, 30, 37, 39, 62, 71, 77, 78, 79, 81, 82

Drug and fluid management 3, 35, 43, 70, 87, 104

Endocrine disorders 61, 104

Gastrointestinal disorders 17, 18, 19, 20, 46, 47, 48, 50, 51, 52, 58

Haematological disorders 91, 92

Infectious disease 1, 6, 7, 15, 20, 34, 40, 50, 63, 80, 105, 107

Malignant disease 10, 19, 41, 47, 49, 36, 39, 60, 61, 67, 79, 90, 98, 102

Mobility and independence 16, 75, 83, 103

Neurological disease 12, 22, 28, 31, 42, 80, 85, 97, 100

Nutrition 56, 69, 106

Respiratory system disease 6, 23, 58, 89, 67, 107

Rheumatological and bone disease 4, 15, 23, 25, 32, 57, 63, 65, 68, 72, 73, 74, 76, 108

Trauma and falls 4, 9, 11, 27, 30, 32, 66, 86

Urological and renal disease 24, 34, 41, 42, 96

Vascular disorders 7, 24, 38, 64, 72

Visual loss 26, 93, 94

Abbreviations

AAA — abdominal aortic aneurysm
ACE — angiotensin-converting enzyme
ACE-I — angiotensin-converting enzyme inhibitor
ADH — antidiuretic hormone
ADL — activities of daily living
A II RA — angiotensin II receptor antagonist
AIDS — acquired immunodeficiency syndrome
ALT — alanine aminotransferase
AMD — age-related macular degeneration
AMTS — Abbreviated Mental Test Score
ANCA — antineutrophil cytoplasmic antibody
APTT — activated partial thromboplastin time
AST — aspartate aminotransferase
ATP — adenosine triphosphate
BMD — bone mineral density
BMI — body mass index
BP — blood pressure
CCB — calcium channel blocker
CJD — Creuzfeldt–Jakob disease
CK — creatine kinase
CMV — cytomegalovirus
CNS — central nervous system
COPD — chronic obstructive pulmonary disease
CREST — calcinosis, Raynaud's, oesophageal involvement, sclerodactyly, telangioectasia
CRP — C-reactive protein
CSF — cerebrospinal fluid
CT — computed tomography
CVA — cerebrovascular accident
DEXA — dual energy X-ray absorptiometry
DNA — deoxyribonucleic acid
DVT — deep vein thrombosis
ECG — electrocardiogram
ECT — electroconvulsive therapy
EEG — electroencephalogram
ERCP — endoscopic retrograde cholangio-pancreatography
ESR — erythrocyte sedimentation rate

FAB — Frontal Assessment Battery
FEV1 — forced expiratory volume in 1 second
FVC — forced vital capacity
GCS — Glasgow Coma Scale
GDS — Geriatric Depression Scale
GFR — glomerular filtration rate
GI — gastrointestinal
GIT — gastrointestinal tract
GP — general practitioner
HbAlc — haemoglobin Alc
HDL — high density lipoprotein
HIV — human immunodeficiency virus
HLA — human leukocyte antigen
HRT — hormone replacement therapy
IgA (G) (M) — immunoglobulin A (G) (M)
INR — international normalized ratio
ISH — isolated systolic hypertension
IVU — intravenous urogram
JVP — jugular venous pressure
LACI — lacunar infarct
LDL — low density lipoprotein
MCH — mean cell haemoglobin
MCV — mean cell volume
MGUS — monoclonal gammopathy of undetermined (uncertain) significance
MI — myocardial infarction
MMSE — Mini-mental State Examination
MR — magnetic resonance
MRC — Medical Research Council
MRI — magnetic resonance imaging
MRSA — methicillin-resistant *Staphylococcus aureus*
MSSU — mid stream specimen of urine
MTP — metatarso-phalangeal
NIHSS — National Institutes of Health Stroke Scale
NPH — normal pressure hydrocephalus
NSAID — nonsteroidal anti-inflammatory drug
OA — osteoarthritis

OGD — oesophagogastro-duodenoscopy
PACI — partial anterior circulation infarct
PAH — pulmonary artery hypertension
PEG — percutaneous endoscopic gastrostomy
PET — positron emission tomography
PLMS — periodic limb movement during sleep
POCI — posterior circulation infarct
PSA — prostate-specific antigen
PXE — pseudo-xanthoma elasticum
RA — rheumatoid arthritis
RBC — red blood cell
REM — rapid eye movement
rTPA — recombinant tissue plasminogen activator
SHEP — systolic hypertension in the elderly programme
SIADH — syndrome of inappropriate secretion of antidiuretic hormone
SLE — systemic lupus erythematosus
SMD — senile macular degeneration
SS — systemic sclerosis
SSRI — selective serotonin reuptake inhibitor
SYST-EUR — systolic hypertension in Europe
TACI — total anterior circulation infarct
TB — tuberculosis
TENS — transcutaneous electrical nerve stimulation
TIA — transient ischaemic attack
TIBC — total iron binding capacity
TNF — tumour necrosis factor
TSH — thyroid stimulating hormone
T3 — triiodothyronine
UK — United Kingdom
UTI — urinary tract infection
ZN — Ziehl–Neelsen

Patient 1

An 82-year-old woman was referred to hospital by her GP as an emergency. She had been acutely confused for 4 days. Prior to that she had complained of a headache for about 1 week and had had at least two rigors. About 1 month before that she had suffered a severe upper respiratory tract infection and was diagnosed by her GP as having frontal sinusitis. Her previous medical history included diet-controlled diabetes mellitus, hypertension, gout, and intermittent depression. Her medication consisted of slow-release diltiazem 120 mg/day, allopurinol 300 mg and citalopram 20 mg at night.

On examination she was found to have a body temperature of 38.2°C and was clearly disorientated in time and place. An attempted AMTS gave a result of 4/10. Her heart rate was 100 bpm and regular, BP 150/90 mmHg. Examination of the cardiovascular system, respiratory system, and abdomen was otherwise normal. CNS examination was difficult because of the delirium but it was noted that she had an extensor plantar reflex on the right.

---

1 List the most important differential diagnoses.

---

2 Which of the following investigations was most likely to provide firm diagnostic information?
A Plain radiography of the skull to show the air sinuses.
B Blood cultures.
C Plain chest radiograph.
D CT head scan.
E Nasopharyngeal bacteriology swab.

Investigations (normal range)

Haemoglobin 15.5 g/dL (11.5–16)
MCV 86 fL (80–96)
Total white cell count 28.2 × 10^9/L (4–11)
Neutrophil count 25.5 × 10^9/L (1.5–7)
ESR 62 mm/h (<30)
Serum sodium 144 mmol/L (137–144)
Serum potassium 4.1 mmol/L (3.5–4.9)
Serum urea 10.1 mmol/L (2.5–7.5)
Serum creatinine 94 μmmol/L (60–110)
Liver function tests and bone chemistry all normal

---

3 The most likely explanation for this patient's raised serum urea was:
A Mild chronic renal failure.
B Dehydration.
C Urate nephropathy.
D An adverse drug reaction.
E A hypercatabolic state.

Patient 2

An 84-year-old woman presented with a left hemiparesis. On examination she was found to have the abnormality below (**2a, 2b**). This was a new sign.

---

1 Which best describes the overall diagnosis?
A Hemispheric stroke.
B Weber's syndrome.
C Foville's syndrome.
D Lateral medullary syndrome.
E Brainstem stroke.

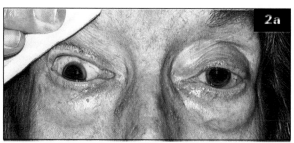

2a Facial appearance of patient.

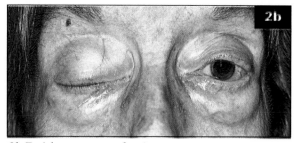

2b Facial appearance of patient.

Patient 1 Answers

1 The most important differential diagnosis in this case is a cerebral abscess. This is supported by the delirium, abnormal neurological findings, headache, high white cell count, and preceding history of a severe upper respiratory tract infection with sinusitis. Other diagnoses to be considered include an aggressive cerebral tumour, though the high white cell count would not be expected in that condition, and severe persisting bacterial sinusitis, which could cause a delirium and a leukocytosis but would not result in an extensor plantar response. Of course, in an elderly person, mixed pathology always needs to be considered.

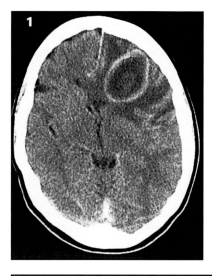

1 CT head scan showing a cerebral abscess.

> **2 D** CT head scan.

A CT head scan is most likely to provide definitive information in this clinical context. A cerebral abscess typically causes a mass lesion with ring enhancement after the injection of contrast, and a substantial amount of surrounding cerebral oedema. An example of this can be seen in Figure 1. CT head scanning also enables an accurate view of the air sinuses of the skull and will also help to rule out other important differential diagnoses such as cerebral tumour. Blood cultures should be performed in such a case because, if positive, they provide useful information to guide antibacterial treatment. Plain radiographs of the skull to outline the air sinuses would probably show a persisting degree of sinus mucosal oedema and secretions but would not help to differentiate the diagnosis further.

> **3 B** Dehydration.

The patient has been acutely confused and febrile for several days. Under such conditions elderly patients are particularly prone to become dehydrated. The slightly high urea accompanied by a creatinine that is still within the normal range and haemoglobin and sodium levels towards the top of the normal range are all consistent with a moderately dehydrated state. The patient might also be hypercatabolic and the increased nitrogen turnover under those conditions can contribute to a high serum urea. The patient's drug therapy does not include any medication expected to cause renal impairment. There is a history of gout that could cause some background renal impairment or indeed, be the result of such a condition, though that is less likely, in this context, than dehydration to be the reason for the raised urea.

Tutorial

Cerebral abscess is not a common condition but it is treatable and the consequences of delayed treatment are catastrophic. Elderly patients are particularly likely to present with delirium and falls and the diagnosis can be clouded by co-pathologies. The typical symptoms are those described in this case. The neurological signs depend on the position of the abscess. A cerebral abscess can result from haematogenous spread of bacteria from sepsis in almost any part of the body, though the well-documented most common associations are with sinusitis, lung abscess, bronchiectasis, penetrating head trauma, middle ear infection, severe head and neck skin and subcutaneous sepsis, and infection involving the intracerebral venous sinuses.

Treatment consists of drainage of the abscess when this is surgically feasible (though very small abscesses do not always require this), antibiotic treatment and dexamethasone to suppress the cerebral oedema in the early stages. Antibiotic treatment should be guided, whenever possible, by bacteriological specimens and prevailing sensitivity patterns. Since cerebral abscesses have been described with a very wide range of organisms including Gram-positive, Gram-negative, and anaerobic, it is important to use broad-spectrum treatment if no specific bacterium has been isolated. It is good practice to discuss all cases of cerebral abscess with a neurosurgical team. In some patients the accompanying evidence of infection may be less clear cut, in which case it can be difficult to determine whether a ring-enhancing lesion on CT is due to cerebral abscess or a cerebral tumour. In such cases, a biopsy to sample the lesion is helpful. Because elderly patients with cerebral abscess often have other co-pathologies, it is important to optimize the medical management of those other conditions to improve the chances of a good outcome from treating the abscess.

Patient 2 Answer

1 **B** Weber's syndrome.

The above pictures show a complete right-sided ptosis and the eye is deviated down and laterally, indicating a third cranial nerve palsy. This suggests a lesion in the midbrain (location of the nucleus of the third cranial nerve). The pyramidal tract fibres would not have crossed over at this level and damage to these fibres in the midbrain leads to a contralateral hemiparesis. The combination of these physical signs is known as 'Weber's syndrome'. The most likely aetiology is a cerebrovascular event but alternative pathology such as a midbrain tumour or demyelination can cause the same clinical picture.

Patient 3

An 85-year-old woman was referred to clinic. She had had four falls over the previous 3 months. She had a past history of ischaemic heart disease and OA, predominantly affecting the knees. She was taking co-dydramol when required, with good symptom control. She denied any loss of consciousness, dizziness, or vertigo and claimed that her falls were due to loss of balance. She was an independent woman and managed to carry out her activities of daily living with a little help from her daughter. A MMSE was 27/30. On examination she had early cataracts. The knees were osteoarthritic but no joint instability was identified. There were normal heart sounds with a 10 mmHg drop in systolic BP on standing. On neurological examination there was generalized MRC grade 4/5 muscle weakness but no focal signs. An ECG showed atrial fibrillation with a rate of 84 bpm. A radiograph of the knees showed mild osteoarthritic changes.

1 What is the intervention that is most likely to help reduce this woman's falls?
   A Refer for early cataract surgery.
   B Provide her with a walking stick.
   C Refer her for a knee replacement.
   D Review her medication.
   E Refer for physiotherapy.

2 What would be the most important change to the medication that needs to be considered?
   A Give digoxin.
   B Add warfarin.
   C Start donepezil.
   D Start fludrocortisone.
   E Stop co-dydramol.

Patient 4

A 79-year-old woman presented with a history of frequent falls at home. She had an extensive past medical history including chronic obstructive pulmonary disease, angina, heart failure, OA, and a recent fractured left hip treated by insertion of a dynamic hip screw. She complained of dizziness but no loss of consciousness or vertigo. Her medication consisted of a Combivent inhaler, isosorbide mononitrate, lisinopril, aspirin, and lactulose. On examination she was frail and it was felt that she had a persisting risk of falls.

1 How would you best manage the patient's risk of future fractures?
   A Perform a DEXA scan before starting treatment.
   B Prescribe calcium supplementation daily.
   C Prescribe calcium and vitamin D3 daily.
   D Prescribe risedronate weekly and calcium/vitamin D3 daily.
   E Prescribe strontium ranelate with calcium daily.

Patient 3 Answers

1 E Refer for physiotherapy.

2 B Add warfarin.

There is evidence that physiotherapy can reduce the frequency of falls in patients with limb weakness. In the history there is nothing to suggest that there was any significant visual impairment so cataract surgery is not indicated at this stage. The walking stick may be helpful but there is no experimental evidence that this should be a routine intervention. The patient does not have arthritis severe enough to warrant a knee replacement. She may benefit from a change in medication to take alternative analgesics such as a NSAID. Alternatively, one can consider a corticosteroid joint injection. Reviewing her medication is an important part of her management. Patients taking more than four medications are more likely to have falls. In addition co-dydramol does have sedating side-effects that might predispose to falls. However, in this case the medication does not seem to be causing significant side-effects and therefore changing it is unlikely to reduce her falls.

Physiotherapy for muscle strengthening, and gait and balance training, have been shown in various clinical trials that included elderly community dwelling females to be effective at reducing falls. This, therefore, is the intervention most likely to be effective in this case.

Digoxin is useful to control the ventricular rate in patients with atrial fibrillation. It has no role in chemically cardioverting the patient or maintaining sinus rhythm. This patient has a controlled ventricular rate therefore digoxin is not required. The patient has nonrheumatic atrial fibrillation; this increases the risk of stroke by about four times. Warfarin has been shown to substantially reduce this risk. This is a difficult decision and the benefit to patients of prescribing warfarin must outweigh the risk of having further falls, with consequent severe bleeding, while on warfarin. This therapeutic dilemma should be discussed with the patient who needs to make an informed decision whenever possible, and the outcome of such a decision should be recorded. This patient has mild cognitive impairment, though based on current recommendations, she would not be thought to warrant an antidementia drug. Postural hypotension is deemed significant if there is a 20 mmHg drop in systolic and a 10 mmHg drop in diastolic BP. The postural hypotension demonstrated in this case was less than that. Another important consideration is that fludrocortisone is not a first line therapy for postural hypotension and, if used, should be carefully monitored because of the possible side-effects it can cause, particularly those due to salt and water retention. Co-dydramol causes drowsiness as a side-effect but there is nothing to suggest that this was the case in the patient described.

Patient 4 Answer

1 D   Prescribe risedronate weekly and calcium/ vitamin D3 daily.

Although a DEXA scan is the investigation of choice to make a diagnosis of osteoporosis, in this case it is neither necessary (because she has had a low-impact fracture) nor appropriate in view of her age and frailty (there are no agreed normal values for such patients), and the OA can interfere with the scan result. Guidelines by the Royal College of Physicians (4) state that patients who have had fractures and are osteopenic (T score of -1 to -2.5) should be treated for osteoporosis. This patient's osteoporosis risk factor status makes her almost certainly at least osteopenic. As she had a fragility fracture she would qualify for treatment, making the DEXA scan unnecessary. Calcium alone has not been shown to be effective at reducing hip fractures. Calcium and vitamin D3 combined has been shown to be effective as primary prevention, though recent studies have failed to show any benefit in the secondary reduction of fractures. Bisphosphonates have been shown to be effective at reducing hip fractures. They are normally prescribed in conjunction with calcium and vitamin D3. A once weekly preparation is much more convenient. Patients are probably more likely to be compliant with a weekly bisphosphonate. Strontium is useful for patients unable to take a bisphosphonate. It causes a predisposition to thromboembolism so is currently not regarded as a first line choice.

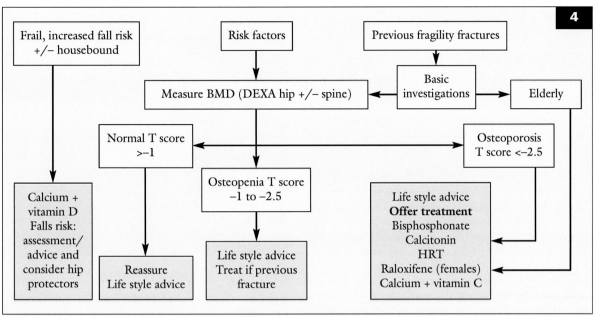

4 Algorithm for the management of known or suspected osteoporosis. (Adapted from guidelines of the Royal College of Physicians.)

Patient 5

A 73-year-old man presented in clinic, accompanied by his wife. They had noticed he was increasingly forgetful. On examination he had a MMSE of 24/30. A 'Get up and Go' Test showed marked ataxia. He was noted to be wearing a sheath urinal. A CT head scan performed soon after this initial assessment is shown (**5a**).

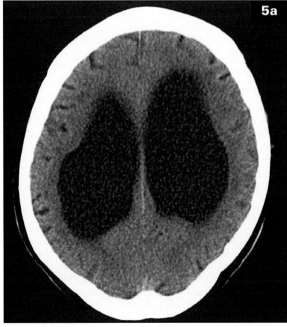

5a CT head scan taken soon after initial assessment.

1 What is usually the first clinical sign of this disorder?
  A Gait disturbance.
  B Urinary incontinence.
  C Faecal incontinence.
  D Dementia.
  E Hemiparesis.

Patient 5 Answer

> 1 A Gait disturbance.

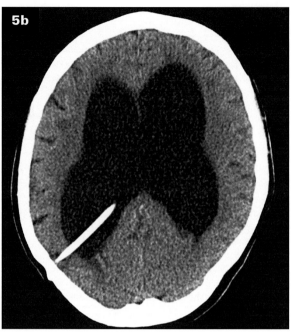

5b

The history and CT scan appearance suggest NPH. A gait disorder is frequently the first clinical symptom or sign, with patients showing difficulty in initiating movement. The presentation may be confused with that of an extrapyramidal disorder such as Parkinson's disease. The term gait apraxia is used in NPH but is considered incorrect by some authors, since patients with NPH can exhibit near-normal walking movements when supported. Patients with NPH demonstrate a short-stepped shuffling gait, with postural instability. The mental deterioration observed is frequently mild and is subcortical in nature. Memory problems, poor attention, and slowing of information processing are observed.

Urinary incontinence is usually present in more advanced cases. Patients usually retain awareness of the incontinence except in the very late stages. A CT or MR scan of the brain shows ventriculo-sulcal disproportion. CSF pressures are normal or intermittently raised.

5b CT head scan showing position of a shunt.

Tutorial

First described in 1965, NPH refers to a clinical syndrome consisting of a triad of gait disturbance, dementia, and incontinence, coupled with the demonstration of normal (or intermittently raised) CSF pressures, and radiographic findings of ventriculomegaly.

NPH is a relatively rare cause of dementia, possibly 6% of cases. Identifying NPH is important because it is often treatable. It is commoner in patients over 60 years. Approximately one half of cases are described as idiopathic. In the other 50% of patients, a history of events that can alter CSF flow dynamics exists, such as previous subarachnoid haemorrhage, trauma, meningitis, or surgery. Clinical symptoms arise because of distortion of the corona radiata. Distortion of sacral motor fibres leads to gait disturbance and incontinence while distortion of the periventricular limbic system causes dementia.

The natural course of NPH is one of continuing cognitive and motor decline, akinetic mutism, and eventual death. This prognosis has probably been improved by the tendency towards surgical intervention since the first description of NPH by Hakim and Adams in 1965, though there are no randomized trials comparing surgery with no surgery. Treatment consists of the insertion of a ventriculo-peritoneal shunt (**5b**). One third of patients improve; in one third, symptom progression is arrested; and one third continue to deteriorate. The complication rate is also approximately one third. Highly selected patients presenting with NPH of known aetiology, an appropriate clinical picture, and ventriculo-sulcal disproportion have a 50–70% favourable response to a shunt, giving a benefit to harm ratio of 3:1. In patients having idiopathic NPH the ratio is less favourable at 1.7:1.

Patient 6

An 89-year-old man was referred to hospital as an urgent outpatient. He had presented to his GP about 10 weeks before complaining of a loss of appetite, weight loss, and cough. Initially, his GP treated him with a 10-day course of doxycycline for a suspected chest infection. There was no improvement with that treatment. His GP performed a chest radiograph that showed shadowing in the left mid zone. Further treatment was given with amoxicillin and some improvement was reported though, after another 3 weeks or so, the patient had again deteriorated. He had a 40 pack-year smoking history and had worked for 1 year as a young man in a coal mine. There was no history of travel outside the UK in the past 20 years, though he had served as a soldier in Burma in World War II. His previous medical history consisted of a peptic ulcer for which he had received a vagotomy and partial gastrectomy in 1965, OA of the knees, and Ménière's disease.

His medication consisted of omeprazole 20 mg daily, paracetamol 1 g as required, and betahistine 8 mg three times daily. In the Outpatient Department further detailed history-taking revealed several episodes of night sweating in the preceding 2 weeks, a continued cough with the production of small amounts of white sputum and an exercise tolerance now limited to about 100 m on the flat. Physical examination revealed a pulse of 80 bpm regular, BP 135/84 mmHg, and no other abnormalities on examination of the cardiovascular system. Abdominal examination revealed a rather scaphoid, cachectic abdomen and an old scar, but was otherwise normal. His respiratory rate was 18 per minute at rest. Expansion was reduced and there was loss of hepatic and cardiac dullness. Coarse crackles were heard in the left lung at the base and mid zone laterally. There were no abnormal neurological signs.

Spirometry performed about 8 weeks previously had shown a moderate obstructive defect. A chest radiograph was performed (**6**).

Investigations (normal range)

Haemoglobin 12.2 g/dL (13–18)
MVC 84 fL (80–96)
Total white cell count 8.2 × 10⁹/L (4–11)
Neutrophil count 6.2 × 10⁹/L (1.5–7)
Lymphocyte count 2.1 × 10⁹/L (1.5–4)
ESR 96 mm/h (<20)
Serum sodium 137 mmol/L (137–144)
Serum potassium 3.9 mmol/L (3.5–4.9)
Serum urea 3.1 mmol/L (2.5–7.5)
Serum creatinine 82 μmol/L (60–110)
Serum albumin 35 g/L (37–49)
Random plasma glucose 5.2 mmol/L (3–6)
Routine liver function tests were otherwise
  normal

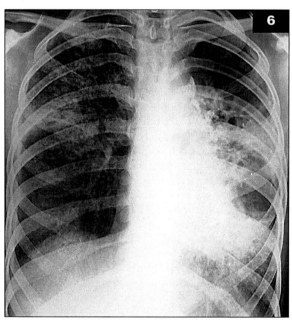

6 Chest radiograph taken at the time of assessment.

1 List the differential diagnoses.

2 Which of the following was the most likely diagnosis in this patient?
   A Bronchogenic carcinoma.
   B Community-acquired pneumonia.
   C Mycoplasma pneumonia.
   D Pulmonary tuberculosis.
   E Coal miner's pneumoconiosis.

3 The patient was admitted to hospital for further investigation about 1 week later and it was found that his serum sodium had fallen to 129 mmol/L. The most important next step in the assessment of this change was:
   A Serum ADH assay.
   B 24-hr urinary sodium loss estimation.
   C Measurement of serum and urine osmolality.
   D A demeclocycline response test.
   E A short Synacthen test.

Patient 6 Answers

1 The most important differential diagnoses in this case are infection (particularly unresolving pyogenic pneumonia and TB) and intrapulmonary malignancy. The relatively abrupt onset, febrile symptoms, and increased sputum production suggests infection and the lack of sustained response to standard antibiotic treatment increases the likelihood of more unusual infections such as TB. The normal total white cell count is also against pyogenic infection, though in older people leukocyte responses are sometimes attenuated, even in acute pneumonia. With the history of exposure to cigarette smoke, the possibility of such a patient having intrapulmonary malignancy is, of course, increased. Other differentials are uncommon and include a wide range of unusual infections, and some patients with the more aggressive forms of pulmonary fibrosis can present in this manner.

3 C Measurement of serum and urine osmolality.

It is likely that this patient has inappropriate ADH secretion in response to intrapulmonary infection. If the plasma osmolality is low in the presence of a high or normal urine osmolality, that will support the diagnosis. The sodium response to demeclocycline in such cases can be useful information, though it should not be employed to establish a diagnosis of inappropriate ADH secretion at this early stage of assessment. There are no other features of Addison's disease so it would be premature at this stage to perform a short Synacthen test, though that would be a reasonable approach if the hyponatraemia persists and inappropriate ADH secretion has been ruled out.

2 D Pulmonary tuberculosis.

The most likely diagnosis, taking into account the clinical history and the chest radiograph appearance is pulmonary TB. However, it is not possible to be certain of this without further investigation. The patient did not have prolonged coal-face exposure so coal miner's pneumoconiosis is extremely unlikely and in any case it would not be expected to present acutely. Unresolving pyogenic infection is a possibility in this context, though the presence of clear sputum with slight blood staining would be unusual in that case. Mycoplasma pneumonia is an acute condition and it would be unlikely to have persisted for so long, particularly after the patient had had a course of doxycycline. Similarly, respiratory syncytial virus would not normally be expected to cause pneumonia with focal consolidation or such a persistent clinical picture.

Tutorial

Pulmonary TB is not uncommon in the UK. High-risk groups include newly arrived immigrants who have come to the UK from areas with a high prevalence of TB and their close contacts, patients with any form of immunosuppression, particularly HIV/AIDS, and elderly people in whom cell-mediated immunity is often impaired compared with younger adults. It is thought that such elderly people may have had dormant TB for many years, and that this reactivates when T-lymphocyte surveillance wanes and suppression of the latent infection becomes inadequate. It is therefore not unusual to make the diagnosis of pulmonary TB in an elderly person who has had no contact with a known sufferer. Once the diagnosis has been considered, it should be investigated and treated in the same way as would be the case for a younger patient. Examination of the sputum by ZN staining and culture is an important first step and in florid open cases will provide all the information required. The chance of obtaining positive specimens is increased by performing bronchoscopy with washings. Tuberculin skin testing is of little or no value in this context. If there is a strong suspicion of TB, treatment should be started even if there is no definite bacteriological confirmation. Treatment should be co-ordinated and guided by a department specializing in the management of TB.

Patient 7

An 82-year-old woman was sent to the hospital as an emergency complaining of shortness of breath, cough, and production of greenish-brown sputum. The symptoms had been present with increasing severity for about 8 days. In the 2 days before admission she had also fainted on standing and had had a fall after rising from a chair. Her husband reported that several episodes of confusion, lasting about half an hour, had also occurred in the past 48 hours. After admission she spontaneously complained of a sharp, knife-like pain in the chest anteriorly and on the left side laterally; the pain was made worse by deep inspiration and coughing. On examination she had a body temperature of 38.2°C, pulse 110 per minute and BP 115/70 mmHg. The heart sounds were normal and cardiac apex difficult to locate. The jugular venous pressure was not raised. Her respiratory rate was 24 per minute and coarse lung crackles were heard at both lung bases and in the left mid zone laterally. Bedside examination of the sputum showed fairly copious greenish-brown sputum that the patient was finding easy to expectorate.

---

1 Describe the abnormalities present on the chest radiograph.

---

2 On the basis of the information available, the most likely reason for this patient's relatively low BP is:
A Dehydration.
B Hypoxia.
C Left ventricular failure.
D Sympathetic neuropathy.
E Sepsis.

Investigations (normal range)

Haemoglobin 10.9 g/dL (11.5–16.5)
Total white cell count 16.5 × 10^9/L (4–11)
Neutrophil count 13.8 × 10^9/L (1.5–7)
ESR 79 mm/h (<30)
Serum sodium, potassium, urea, and
    creatinine all within the normal range
Arterial blood gas analysis revealed:
PO_2 9.6 kPa (11.3–12.6)
PCO_2 4.9 kPa (4.7–6)
pH 7.41 (7.36–7.44)
Gram staining of sputum showed very large
    numbers of *Staphylococcus aureus*
    (subsequent culture revealed the organism
    to be sensitive to flucloxacillin)
Blood cultures 4 bottles negative
Admission chest radiograph (**7a**)

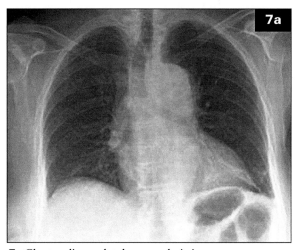

7a Chest radiograph taken on admission.

The patient was treated with intravenous flucloxacillin and became afebrile. At this stage the working diagnosis was staphylococcal pneumonia. However, her condition relapsed and she became breathless again, and a further chest radiograph was taken (**7b**). A sample of the pleural effusion revealed heavily bloodstained fluid. Her BP had fallen to 95/50 mmHg, though there were no other new physical signs in the heart or chest.

---

3 At this stage the best choice of further investigation to establish the underlying pathology was:
A Ventilation–perfusion isotope lung scan.
B CT scan of the thorax.
C Cardiac catheterization.
D Thoracic ultrasound scan.
E Left lateral chest radiograph.

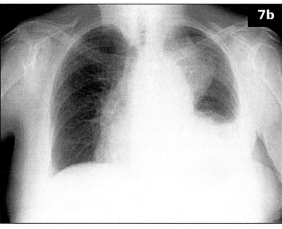

7b Follow-up chest radiograph taken 10 days later.

Patient 7 Answers

1 There is slight unfolding of the thoracic aorta, which is not uncommon in patients of this age. At this stage it was thought that this degree of aortic distortion was of no particular clinical importance and was most probably due to degenerative change in the wall of the aorta. There was slight coarsening of the bronchovascular markings and some possible early inflammatory shadowing at the left lung base. Other than that, there were no major abnormalities. The chest radiograph (**7a**) certainly did not show the abnormalities usually associated with staphylococcal pneumonia, such as patchy consolidation with cavitation. The cardiothoracic ratio on this radiograph was normal.

---

2 E Sepsis.

Sepsis was the most likely reason for the tendency to hypotension. There was good evidence of a septic process in that the patient was febrile, had a neutrophil leukocytosis, a high ESR and evidence of respiratory tract infection with a specific organism. The patient was not sufficiently hypoxic for that to be the cause of hypotension and she was not acidotic. There was no evidence of dehydration on the blood investigations. The chest radiograph showed no radiological evidence of heart failure and there were no physical signs to suggest heart failure; the tachycardia was in proportion to the rise in body temperature. There was no evidence in the clinical history or on physical examination to point towards a sympathetic neuropathy, which in any case would normally cause postural hypotension, rather than a persistent supine hypotension.

---

3 B CT scan of the thorax.

The follow-up chest radiograph (**7b**) shows a left-sided pleural effusion and probable expansion of the intrathoracic aorta that had occurred over a very short period of time. The best option to capture all of the underlying pathology was to perform a CT scan of the thorax. This enabled imaging of the heart, great vessels, lungs, pericardium, and the pleural fluid. Little would have been gained by performing a left lateral chest radiograph in this case. Chest ultrasound would only have been helpful to confirm the presence of pleural fluid and to guide sampling. It would not provide any further information about the heart and great vessels and, in any case, pleural fluid had already been sampled in this patient. There is no convincing indication for ventilation–perfusion lung scanning. By this stage it was clear that other pathologies were more likely to be the explanation for the patient's hypotension and tachycardia, and the degree of hypoxia was not that which would be expected in a pulmonary embolism large enough to cause this degree of hypotension. Cardiac catheterization would certainly give a detailed outline of the cardiac chambers and vessels, though it would provide no information about the pericardium or pleural cavity. Furthermore, because the nature of the aortic pathology was not clear at this stage, there was a risk that an interventional procedure could worsen the patient's clinical state by precipitating an overt rupture of the aorta.

CT of the thorax was performed (**7c**). There was abnormal dilatation of the aorta with some leakage of probable blood into the pericardium and pleural cavity. A mass lesion eroding from the aorta can be seen, and it was thought this was probably a mycotic aneurysm. Transoesophageal echocardiography confirmed those findings and also demonstrated an intact aortic valve. The patient was referred for urgent cardiac surgery and had the successful replacement of her aortic arch with a prosthetic graft. The resected surgical specimen revealed a mycotic aneurysm and adjacent para-aortic abscess containing *Staphylococcus aureus* of the same strain isolated from the sputum.

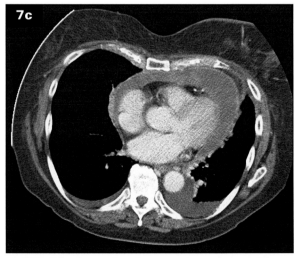

7c CT of the thorax showing mycotic aneurysm of the ascending aorta and pericardial fluid.

Tutorial (Patient 7)

This patient illustrates two very important issues. Firstly, whenever a patient is found to have significant staphylococcal sepsis, the clinician should be vigilant for the possible presence of the same organism elsewhere in the body. Seeding of staphylococci can occur almost anywhere and in elderly patients it is particularly important to think of this process as a possible cause for septic discitis, septic arthritis, osteomyelitis and, as in this case, mycotic aneurysms. Secondly, this patient had no known predisposing risk factors for staphylococcal sepsis, so the absence of a history of recent surgery or instrumentation, immunosuppression, or other predisposing conditions such as diabetes, should not deter the clinician from looking for infection with *Staphylococcus aureus*. Mycotic aneurysms in the aorta are not common but are amenable to treatment if prompt action is taken. It is thought that the aortic wall is predisposed to bacterial invasion if it is damaged by degenerative processes, such as atherosclerosis, or other inflammatory conditions such as syphilitic aortitis or spondylitic aortitis. Factors in favour of a good outcome from surgery in this patient were her preceding good functional status, lack of co-pathologies, normal renal function, normal left ventricular function, and preservation of the aortic valve.

Patient 8

A 79-year-old female's neighbour contacted the local health centre because she was worried about the elderly woman's behaviour. The GP called and found the patient to be seemingly rational but unable to give a good reason for the fact that she was hoarding a vast number of newspapers and milk bottles, to the extent that one of the ceiling joists of her rented council house had cracked from the weight. The patient was fully mobile, with a normal 'Get up and Go' Test, a Barthel ADL index score of 20/20, a MMSE score of 28/30, normal frontal lobe tests, and a normal score on the GDS. She was a retired music teacher who lived alone and had no family. She had had very little contact with her GP over the preceding years and took no medications. The house was untidy and squalid, with a lot of stale food, dirty dishes, and unwashed clothes. All the services were functioning. Physical examination of the patient revealed no abnormalities, though there was evidence of weight loss. There were no psychotic symptoms and her piano playing was fluent and precise.

The patient's doctor arranged for blood to be taken for basic haematology, renal function, liver function, thyroid function, blood glucose, and ESR, all of which were normal. On a follow-up visit the ceiling appeared to be on the verge of collapse, though the patient was not keen to do anything about it despite admitting to the danger.

1 The best course of action at this stage is:
 A Remove the patient from the house to a hospital by use of the Mental Health Act.
 B Ask a psychiatrist to provide a second opinion by doing a domiciliary visit.
 C Persuade the patient to leave the house and go into temporary emergency local authority accommodation.
 D Order the house to be vacated by use of the Public Health Act.
 E Get a builder in to shore up the ceiling.

2 Which is the most likely diagnosis?
 A Atypical depression.
 B Fronto-temporal dementia.
 C Early Alzheimer's disease.
 D Diogenes syndrome.
 E Obsessive-compulsive disorder.

3 How should the patient be managed?

Patient 8 Answers

---

1 C Persuade the patient to leave the house and go into temporary emergency local authority accommodation.

---

2 D Diogenes syndrome.

There is clearly a danger of a ceiling collapse. This poses a risk to the patient and to any staff or friends who enter the house. Ideally, the patient should have the danger explained and be asked to leave the house immediately, but voluntarily, and go to an appropriate temporary dwelling. This might be the house of a relative or friend, but could be accommodation arranged urgently by social services. There are no grounds to suspect that the patient has a mental illness that would justify a compulsory admission to hospital under the provisions of the Mental Health Act; though that option would be suitable in similar cases when the evidence of significant dementia, depression, or psychosis is clear and the patient needs to be placed in a safe environment as a 'duty of care' to a patient who lacks mental capacity. A psychiatric opinion can be very helpful under such circumstances, and would be an option to be considered in the case described, though the risk from structural failure of the house was deemed to be urgent, so there was no time to take that approach. If the patient refused to vacate the house despite the clear danger, and especially if the patient denied the danger, that would justify a provisional assumption of lack of capacity in which case the patient could be removed, in her 'best interests'. In a less urgent example of structural failure of a building, a person refusing to vacate can be compelled by a magistrate to leave the premises in the interests of public safety.

Shoring up the ceiling in these circumstances would probably be part of the immediate site plan, but would have to be done after the patient has left the house.

The clinical presentation in this patient is highly suggestive of the Diogenes syndrome. This is characterized by a lapse into hoarding, squalor, and self-neglect and is usually seen in elderly people living alone. The self-neglect can be extreme and life-threatening. About half of patients with this presentation have some degree of depression, dementia, or a history of psychosis, though the remainder have no evidence of a formal psychiatric condition (as in the case presented), and in any case depression and dementia are so common in older people that some of the association is likely to be coincidence. It is more commonly seen in women. There is a tendency for the patients to have higher than average intelligence and many have obsessive-compulsive traits or followed professions requiring attention to detail.

The other options in the question include some of the important differential diagnoses, though there was no evidence in the case described to make any of them more likely than the Diogenes syndrome. It is important to exclude depression because of the obvious benefits of treatment. Some patients with dementia show a drift into self-neglect and in some there can be benefit from drugs such as galantamine.

3 For the patient described there was a need for her to vacate the house. In most cases that would not be an urgent issue. If the degree of self-neglect is very severe there is a need for hospital-based treatments to assure nutrition and hydration and to assess the patient's physical state under close scrutiny, and to diagnose and treat any co-morbidities. Further mental state assessment can also be done. In some cases, the patient can be persuaded to allow agencies to clear the hoarded items and clean up the residence, after which regular help to manage the dwelling and to provide food and drink can result in an effective long-term coping strategy. That is the best option for patients with mental capacity. For those who lack capacity, a similar regimen can be effective, though if there is great physical or mental frailty it is more realistic to advise residential care. Associated medical and psychiatric disorders must be treated. There is some evidence of benefit from cognitive behaviour therapy for the Diogenes syndrome, though long-term supervision and practical help appear to be the most effective interventions.

Patient 9

An 85-year-old man with a history of falls presented to the Accident and Emergency Department after having sustained another fall. He complained of right-sided chest pain. A chest radiograph on admission is shown (**9a**). Twenty four hours later he still complained of a painful chest and was noted to be short of breath with an oxygen saturation of 85%. A chest radiograph during this symptomatic deterioration is shown (**9b**).

1 What does the radiograph on admission show?

2 What is the likely cause of the patient's symptomatic deterioration?
A Pneumonia.
B Pleural effusion.
C Complicated pacemaker insertion.
D Pulmonary embolism.
E Haemothorax.

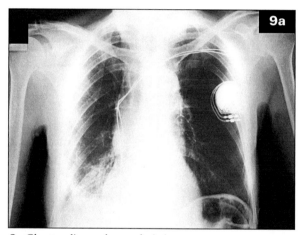

9a Chest radiograph on admission.

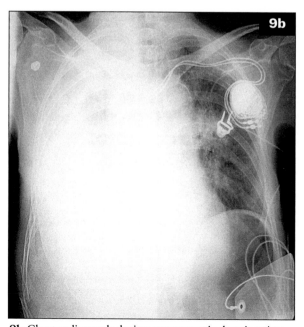

9b Chest radiograph during symptomatic deterioration.

Patient 9 Answers

1 There is a pacemaker visible with a hyperinflated chest. There is shadowing visible in the right lower lobe. At this stage the shadowing has a wide differential diagnosis.

<hr/>

2 E Haemothorax.

<hr/>

The second radiograph shows a fractured rib (**9c**, arrow). This was almost certainly present at the time of his first film but was not clearly visible. The sudden deterioration in the appearance of the right hemi thorax suggests a complication from his rib fracture, most likely a haemothorax.

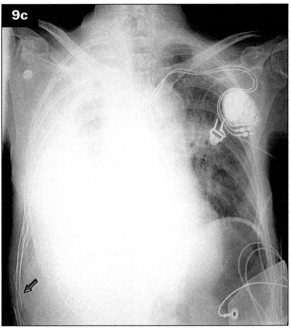

9c Chest radiograph showing a rib fracture (arrow).

Tutorial

The frequency of rib fractures rises with age due to brittleness of the chest wall. In elderly or chronically ill patients, rib fractures can occur with severe coughing or hard straining. Older women have more rib fractures than men. Nontraumatic rib fractures are commoner among older women who also have osteoporosis. They can carry significant morbidity and mortality. Patients with one or two rib fractures are reported to have a 5% admission mortality rate and patients with seven or more fractures have around 30% admission mortality rate. Lung-related morbidity rates of patients with multiple rib fractures are 13–69% in various observational studies. Spontaneous pathological fractures may occur in metastatic disease and in severe metabolic disease such as hyperparathyroidism.

Rib fractures cause pain; this compromises ventilation and effective coughing as patients instinctively try to limit chest wall movements. This impairment may result in atelectasis, retained secretions, and pneumonia. Multiple rib fractures can cause a flail chest, which can result in ventilatory insufficiency due to ineffective respiratory action. Broken ribs can penetrate the lungs and pleura, resulting in a haemothorax or pneumothorax. Such injuries can also affect the extrapleural space, the mediastinum, the heart and great vessels, the spine, and shoulders. The location of specific rib fractures is an important indicator of related injury.

Table 9a presents advice on how to manage a fractured rib.

Table 9a *Evaluating and managing a fractured rib*

- Gently touch the area of the chest that received the blow, looking for sharp tenderness.
- Ask the injured person to take a deep breath or cough; does he/she feel sharp stabbing pain? If yes, suspect a fractured rib
- Look for additional signs and symptoms:
  - Deformity or discolouration around the chest area; shallow breathing to minimize pain; cyanosis or an elevated respiratory rate. The presence of any of these signs may indicate a fractured rib. (Place one hand on each side of the chest. If one side of the chest rises during inhalation while the other falls, at least three ribs have been broken on the falling side of the chest)
  - Signs of a punctured lung: increased difficulty of breathing; coughing up blood
- Decrease movement on the side of the fracture using one of the following methods: tape the fractured side with four or five pieces of adhesive tape from the sternum to the spine; apply an elastic bandage around the entire chest; use a sling to immobilize the arm against the injured side
- Administer adequate analgesia
- Encourage the injured person to cough frequently, despite the pain, in order to prevent secretions from pooling in the lung and causing pneumonia

Patient 10

An 80-year-old man presented with a 2-month history of falls and an unsteady gait. He had no headaches but complained of a sensation of being off balance when walking that disappeared when sitting. He mentioned occasional arthritic pains but had no other symptoms of note. He was taking co-proxamol regularly. On examination he had an abbreviated mental test score of 10/10. He had early cataracts and some hearing impairment but he claimed that this was long-standing as a consequence of his previous occupation. He had Heberden's and Bouchard's nodes in his hands. There was crepitus in his right knee but no joint instability. His gait was very ataxic but there were no focal neurological signs. He had no drop in his systolic BP on standing and there were no cardiovascular, respiratory, or abdominal findings on examination. CT (**10a**, **10b**) and MR (**10c**) head scans were performed.

1 What do the CT head scans (**10a**, **10b**) show?

2 What does the MR scan (**10c**) show?

3 How would you manage this patient?

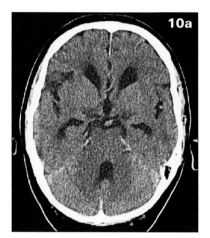

10a Head CT scan taken after initial assessment.

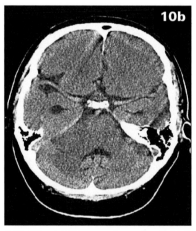

10b Head CT scan taken after initial assessment.

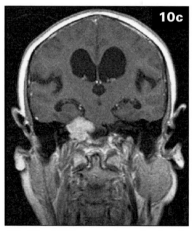

10c Head MR scan taken after head CT scan.

Patient 11

An 85-year-old patient was recovering from pneumonia. He was bed-bound and almost immobile. You were asked to assess his risk of falls before staff started to mobilize him.

1 Which of these was the most appropriate initial assessment?
   A Assess muscle weakness using MRC criteria.
   B Perform a Romberg's Test.
   C Perform a 'Get up and Go' Test.
   D Check his visual acuity.
   E Perform the 'One leg Stand' Test.

Patient 10 Answers

1, 2 The CT scan (**10a**) shows dilatation of the lateral ventricles and marked dilatation of the 4th ventricle. There is a degree of cerebral atrophy consistent with age. The scan in Figure **10b** is taken at the level of the cerebellum and shows displacement and compression of the 4th ventricle. Further imaging of the lesion was required to determine its aetiology. The MR image shows a cerebellopontine angle tumour on the right (**10c**). The scan also shows dilatation of the lateral ventricles.

The patient's presentation was vague with several nonspecific complaints. He had a typical history of disequilibrium, that can be defined as a sensation of unsteadiness or light-headedness while walking that typically disappears when sitting. Disequilibrium is often due to multiple chronic conditions such as visual impairment, drug intoxication, and psychological causes. It is useful to distinguish disequilibrium from vertigo and syncope as an aid to the differential diagnosis.

Vertigo is a sensation of rotation of self or of the surroundings. It is due to peripheral vestibular, central vestibular, or CNS disorders such as ischaemia, infection, or migraine. Syncope is a sudden brief loss of consciousness due to global impairment of the cerebral circulation with spontaneous recovery. It is due to a variety of disorders including cardiovascular and neurological (mainly autonomic) disease.

This case illustrates some of the difficulties associated with assessing elderly patients. The presence of multiple pathology, the atypical presentation of disease, and difficulties with history taking make the process of reaching a diagnosis complicated. There is a need to have a high index of suspicion to home in on the correct diagnosis. In this patient there was considerable overlap between these symptoms. Probably, the most important clue to suggest the need for brain imaging was the severe gait instability.

3 He should be discussed with a neurosurgeon with a view to insertion of a shunt to relieve pressure, or resection of the tumour.

Patient 11 Answer

> **1 C** Perform a 'Get up and Go' Test.

The 'Get up and Go' Test is the test to identify patients at risk of falls recommended by the joint American Geriatrics Society, British Geriatrics Society, and the American Academy of Orthopaedic Surgeons Panel on Falls Prevention. While muscle weakness is an important risk factor for falls it does not provide the best answer in this case. Similarly, the Romberg's test is not a validated test to predict the risk of falls. Though visual acuity is an important part of the physical examination, and poor vision is a risk factor for falls, it is not the best answer in this case. The 'One leg Stand' Test does not exist.

Tutorial

The 'Get up and Go' Test is easily performed. To begin, have the patient sit in a high seat chair with a straight back. The patient may use a walking aid if they normally use one. The following instructions should then be given to the patient.

- Get up without using arm rests if possible.
- Stand still momentarily.
- Walk forward 10 feet (3 m).
- Turn around and walk back to chair.
- Turn and be seated.

The observer must note:
- The patient's sitting balance.
- Transfers from sitting to standing.
- Pace and stability of walking.
- Ability to turn safely without staggering.

Balance function is firstly scored on a five-point scale: 1 = normal; 2 = very slightly abnormal; 3 = mildly abnormal; 4 = moderately abnormal; 5 = severely abnormal. Patient with scores of more than 3 are at risk for falling. However, a judgement has to be made as to whether the patient can do the test safely. A timed version of the test has been described. Timings greater than 10 seconds have a higher risk of falls. The 'Get Up and Go' Test is a very simple test to do, does not require much training, and can easily be done in a busy working environment. It is just as accurate in detecting an abnormal gait, and a risk of falls as a more complex, time consuming gait and balance assessment.

Patient 12

A 90-year-old man was referred for urgent outpatient assessment. He had been feeling well until about 2 months before the referral. Over the following few weeks he had a reduced appetite, lost about 6 kg in weight and had intermittent chills and some night sweats. He called his GP urgently because of pain and tenderness in the skin over the left side of his chest posteriorly and laterally. On examination at that time the GP found no abnormalities other than a degree of tenderness. When seen in the clinic 3 days later the pain was more severe and the patient had noticed a rash (12). The patient had a history of benign prostatic hypertrophy for which he was taking tamsulosin, and hypertension for which he was taking bendroflumethiazide 2.5 mg daily. He had no other significant medical history. Systems review revealed no additional information. On examination he had a body temperature of 37.6°C, pulse 88 bpm regular, heart sounds normal, with no physical signs of heart failure. Examination of the chest revealed a respiratory rate of 14 per minute, visual inspection of the chest showed a rash (12) extending from close to the mid line posteriorly to the mid axillary region in a band-like distribution. Auscultation of the chest was normal, abdominal examination was normal, apart from very loose skin folds suggestive of weight loss.

Investigations (normal range)

Haemoglobin 13.9 g/dL (13–18)
White cell count 12.1 × 10⁹/L (4–11)
Neutrophil count 8.2 × 10⁹/L (1.5–7)
ESR 110 mm/h (<20)
Serum sodium 135 mmol/L (137–144)
Serum potassium 4.6 mmol/L (3.5–4.9)
Serum urea 8.2 mmol/L (2.5–7.5)
Corrected calcium 2.8 mmol/L (2.2–2.6)
Serum albumin 41 g/L (37–47)
Serum alkaline phosphatase 190 units/L (45–105)
Plasma osmolality 290 mosm/kg (278–305)
Urine osmolality 620 mosm/kg (350–1000)

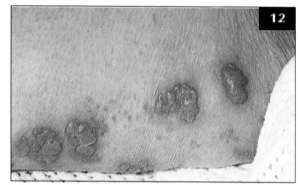

12 The rash identified in clinic.

1 On the basis of the clinical information available, the most important next step in this patient's management is:
   A Treatment with oral acyclovir.
   B Treatment with intravenous broad-spectrum antibiotics.
   C Topical treatment with capsaicin.
   D Pain control using gabapentin.
   E High-dose corticosteroids.

2 The most likely cause of the patient's hyponatraemia is:
   A Low salt intake.
   B Long-term treatment with bendroflumethiazide.
   C Inappropriate secretion of ADH.
   D Senile hyponatraemia.
   E A side-effect of tamsulosin.

3 After settling the acute presenting illness, there were clinical and laboratory indications for further investigation. List the most important differential diagnoses of the underlying pathology.

4 Which of the following investigations is least appropriate in this patient?
   A Plasma protein electrophoresis.
   B PSA.
   C Plain chest radiograph.
   D Convalescent viral antibody titres.
   E Abdominal ultrasound scan.

Patient 12 Answers

1 A Treatment with oral acyclovir.

The patient required treatment immediately with acyclovir or a similar antiviral agent effective against herpes zoster. The mode of presentation and the presence of a vesicular rash in dermatomal distribution were typical of shingles. In some patients pain and/or erythema can precede the eruption of vesicles in the affected dermatome. Antibiotic treatment would be ineffective. Topical capsaicin can be used to manage chronic postherpetic neuralgia though it is contraindicated during the acute attack, at which time it would exacerbate the pain. Similarly, gabapentin can be used for postherpetic neuralgia but does not have an established role in the management of the acute pain during an attack of shingles. High-dose corticosteroids can be used to suppress almost any inflammatory condition though there is no evidence to support the use in the management of shingles. The prompt use of acyclovir at the early vesicular stage reduces the likelihood of prolonged postherpetic neuralgia. In a patient who is otherwise well and is able to swallow, there is no advantage to be gained from giving the acyclovir intravenously. Topical acyclovir has been shown to be effective and is an important part of the management of shingles involving the ophthalmic branch of the trigeminal nerve.

2 B Long-term treatment with bendroflumethiazide.

The most likely reason for the patient's mild hyponatraemia is the treatment with bendroflumethiazide. Sodium intake is rarely sufficiently low to compromise sodium homeostasis in the UK and there were no indications in this patient's history to suggest that that might be the case. The patient's serum and urine osmolalities did not support the diagnosis of inappropriate ADH secretion. The term senile hyponatraemia should be avoided; the majority of elderly people with a hyponatraemic state will have an identifiable underlying cause. Hyponatraemia is not a side-effect of tamsulosin.

3 The background history indicated that the patient had been ill for about 2 months. The presentation to hospital with shingles suggested suppressed cell-mediated immunity. There is some decline in cell-mediated immunity with age and some otherwise healthy individuals will present with shingles as a result of that. In this patient the reduced appetite, weight loss, febrile symptoms and night sweats, very high ESR, and mild hypercalcaemia all suggested serious predisposing pathology. This included myeloma, lymphoma, and carcinoma (possibly with bony metastases). The possibility of chronic infection such as TB or a chronic pyogenic infection must be considered. This differential diagnosis would be a starting point and is by no means exhaustive.

4 D Convalescent viral antibody titres.

In this context the least helpful investigation would have been convalescent viral antibody titres. The nature of the viral infection was known to be herpes zoster in this case and that infection did not explain the preceding 2 months of ill health. The other investigations could all have helped to resolve the differential diagnosis listed in Answer 3 above.

Tutorial

An attack of shingles in an older person should always prompt a search for an underlying predisposing illness, though it must be remembered that the majority of such patients will not have serious underlying pathology. Shingles occurs when dormant herpes zoster viruses in a dorsal nerve root ganglion escape from T-lymphocyte control, replicate, and migrate down nerve axons in the dermatome involved. The virus is identical to that which causes chicken pox and all patients presenting with shingles will have had a clinically obvious or subclinical infection with the virus earlier in life. The most important complications of an attack of shingles are postherpetic neuralgia, blindness due to herpes conjunctivitis or herpes panophthalmitis, and deafness due to eighth cranial nerve involvement (rare). Some patients develop life-threatening complications such as disseminated herpes zoster infection presenting like a severe form of chicken pox, pneumonitis, encephalitis, and meningitis. These complications are usually only seen in patients with severely suppressed immunity.

Patient 13

An 85-year-old man with a history of diabetes mellitus presented to the Accident and Emergency Department within 2 hours of the sudden onset of a right hemiparesis. A CT scan of the brain showed an early infarct in the region of the middle cerebral artery. A full blood count, clotting screen, and renal screen were all normal. His random plasma glucose was 10 mmol/L on admission. An ECG showed sinus rhythm.

1 How should this patient be initially managed?
  A Thrombolysis.
  B Aspirin orally immediately.
  C Dipyridamole orally immediately.
  D Heparin intravenously.
  E Warfarin orally.

Patient 14

This 78-year-old hypertensive and diabetic woman developed sudden onset of loss of vision in the inferior quadrantic area of her left eye. Her symptoms resolved over 2 hours. She had had a similar episode 1 month previously. Fundoscopic examination of the left eye is shown (**14a**). Her BP was 165/90 mmHg with a pulse of 84 bpm and regular. There were no other cardiovascular, respiratory, abdominal, or neurological abnormalities. No carotid bruits were heard. Investigations revealed a random glucose of 10.4 mmol/L.

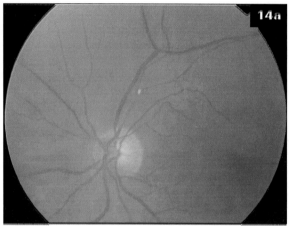

14a Retinal photograph taken at the time of presentation.

1 What is the abnormality seen on the retinal photograph?
  A Retinal detachment.
  B Retinitis pigmentosa.
  C Proliferative diabetic retinopathy.
  D Cholesterol embolus.
  E Acute glaucoma.

2 What further investigation is urgently required?
  A Full blood count.
  B HDL/LDL cholesterol.
  C Ambulatory BP monitor.
  D Carotid doppler.
  E HbA1C.

Patient 13 Answer

> **1 B** Aspirin orally immediately.

This patient presents with a stroke of less than 3 hours duration. Thrombolysis could be considered if the facility is available. However, this man does not satisfy the prevailing criteria on the basis of advanced age and history of diabetes. As the incidence of complications rises significantly above the age of 80 years and in diabetics, on the basis of current recommendations, thrombolysis with rTPA should not be given but aspirin 300 mg immediately, followed by 75 mg daily, is considered to be the best initial management choice.

Inclusion criteria for stroke thrombolysis:
- Clinical signs and symptoms of definite acute stroke.
- Clear time of onset.
- Presentation within 3 hours of onset.
- Haemorrhage excluded by CT scan.
- 18–80 years old.
- NIHSS score >4 to <25.

Exclusion criteria
- Rapidly improving or minor stroke symptoms.
- Stroke or serious head injury within 3 months.
- Major surgery/external heart massage/obstetric delivery within 14 days.
- GI haemorrhage/urinary tract haemorrhage within 21 days.
- History of intracranial haemorrhage, aneurysm, neoplasm, spinal or cranial surgery, or haemorrhagic retinopathy.
- Symptoms suggestive of subarachnoid haemorrhage even if CT normal.
- Systolic BP >185 mmHg and diastolic BP >110 mmHg. (BP reduction to meet criteria not permitted)
- Known clotting disorder.
- Patient on heparin or warfarin.
- Suspected iron deficient anaemia or thrombocytopenia.
- Blood glucose <3 mmol/l or >22 mmol/l.
- Seizure at start of stroke.
- High premorbid dependency.
- Bacterial endocarditis/pericarditis.
- Acute pancreatitis/oesophageal varices/ulcerative GI disease within 3 months/aortic aneurysm/active hepatitis/cirrhosis.
- Prior stroke *and* concomitant diabetes.
- Puncture of noncompressible blood vessel in the last 14 days.

Tutorial

Thrombolysis should be considered if patients present within 3 hours of the onset of symptoms. A CT scan is mandatory before any further decision is taken to thrombolyse or not. Inclusion and exclusion criteria should be strictly adhered to and informed consent should be taken.

Patient 14 Answers

> **1 D** Cholesterol embolus.

> **2 D** Carotid doppler.

The fundus shows a cholesterol embolus along the superior temporal branch of the left retinal artery (**14b**). There is no evidence of retinal detachment, diabetic retinopathy, or cupping from glaucoma. The pigmentary changes in the background are a normal variant and not characteristic of retinitis pigmentosa.

It is important to reduce the overall cardiovascular risk by gaining better control of her BP, diabetes, and cholesterol level. However, at this point in time this patient is at high risk of a full blown stroke and needs urgent carotid dopplers to investigate the possibility of carotid stenosis. She might require carotid surgery if significant stenosis of >75% is identified. As this woman is getting well-documented transient ischaemic attacks she might be a candidate for surgery even at lesser degrees of stenosis.

Tutorial (Patient 14)

As this woman is diabetic she needs tighter BP control. For a patient with cerebrovascular disease and diabetes BP readings of 140/85 mmHg or less should be the target.

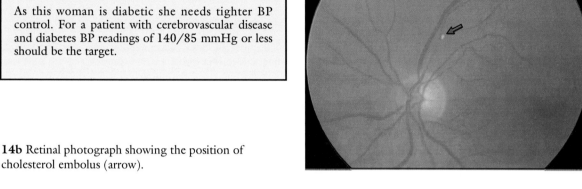

14b Retinal photograph showing the position of cholesterol embolus (arrow).

Patient 15

A 76-year-old man was assessed urgently at his home because he had developed severe mid dorsal back pain for 2 days. He had been discharged from hospital about 4 weeks earlier after emergency surgery for intestinal obstruction due to adhesions. There was a difficult postoperative period in the Intensive Care Unit during which he received fluids, antibiotics, and inotropes through a central venous line. His previous history included diet-controlled diabetes mellitus, hypertension, and benign prostatic hyperplasia. His medication was perindopril 4 mg daily. Examination revealed a distressed man with an oral temperature of 36.8°C, pulse 88 bpm regular, heart sounds normal, BP 150/90 mmHg, respiratory rate 14 per minute. His lung bases were clear on auscultation. Abdominal examination was normal apart from a surgical scar and there were no focal neurological signs. His back pain was too severe for him to be able to roll over in his bed to allow proper physical examination. Opiate analgesia was given and he was readmitted to hospital.

An ECG showed T-wave inversion in the inferior leads but was otherwise normal. The chest radiograph was reported as normal. A radiograph of the dorsal spine showed minor osteophyte formation at several levels and wedging of D12 and L2 vertebrae, though these changes were noted on old radiographs and had not changed. A plasma glucose which was taken in the fasting state shortly after admission was 7.2 mmol/L (3–6), HbA1C 7.5% (3.8–6.4).

Investigations (normal range)

Haemoglobin 10.9 g/dL (13–18)
Total white cell count 11.2 × 10⁹/L (4–11)
Neutrophil count 9.4 × 10⁹/L (1.5–7)
ESR 94 mm/h (<20)
Serum urea 6.1 mmol/L (2.5–7.5)
Serum sodium 139 mmol/L (137–144)
Serum potassium 3.9 mmol/L (3.5–4.9)
Serum albumin 32 g/L (37–49)
Serum bilirubin 18 μmol/L (1–22)
Serum ALT 24 U/L (4–35)
Serum alkaline phosphatase 53 U/L (45–105)
Serum corrected calcium 2.3 mmol/L (2.2–2.6)

1 List the main differential diagnoses for the acute mid line back pain.

2 Which of the following investigations is mostly likely to yield the best diagnostic information?
 A MR scan of the spine.
 B Isotope bone scan.
 C Helical CT of spine.
 D Contrast myelography.
 E Spinal DEXA scan.

3 In this clinical context the most likely diagnosis is:
 A Prolapsed intervertebral disc.
 B Osteoporotic collapse of a vertebra.
 C Metastatic disease.
 D Septic discitis.
 E Osteomyelitis.

Patient 15 Answers

1 In this context the most important differential diagnoses can be arrayed in anatomical terms. Acute bone pain can be caused by fracture, malignancy, or infection. Soft tissue pain may arise from the supporting ligamentous structures of the spine due to trauma, infection, malignancy or noninfective inflammatory disorders. Mid line back pain may also be felt in patients who have paraspinal mass lesions due to malignancy or infection, particularly if there is abscess formation or intense inflammation. A prolapsed intervertebral disc can cause pain locally by direct pressure on ligamentous structures and by impingement on the spinal cord and nerve roots. Penetrating injury as a cause of acute back pain is very unusual in elderly patients but needs to be included, particularly if there is a recent history of local injection therapy close to the source of pain.

---

2 A MR scan of the spine.

An MR scan of the spine. The patient has several features to suggest that a septic process may be present. These include a persisting high ESR, the recent urgent abdominal surgery, and the recent central venous line insertion. MR scanning will show the presence of inflammation in intevertebral discs and bone and will pick up paraspinal inflammatory conditions. Therefore, in this particular case, MR scanning is the best choice. An isotope bone scan will provide information of abnormal uptake to bone in conditions such as fracture, malignancy, and infection, though it will not provide information about soft tissue inflammation. In patients with septic discitis there is often enhanced uptake in the vertebrae on either side of the affected disc. Helical CT scanning of the spine will detect most pathologies but is less sensitive than MR at picking up active inflammation, particularly when there has been no overt destruction of anatomical structures. There is now virtually no indication for contrast myelography. DEXA scanning is used for semiquantitative assessment of osteoporosis and would not provide useful information in this patient.

---

3 D Septic discitis.

A number of clues make septic discitis the most likely diagnosis in this patient. Firstly, the severe back pain with high ESR and recent central venous cannulation. Bacteria can be seeded to various parts of the body when a central cannula is in place and cause a deep infection that takes some time to present clinically. Staphylococcal infection is the most likely. A prolapsed intervertebral disc is a possibility, though these usually occur in the lumbar and sacral regions and are unusual in the dorsal spine. Osteoporotic collapse of a vertebra can be excruciatingly painful and there may be minimal changes on plain radiography. The existing crush fractures in this patient's case are in the wrong part of the spine to account for the pain. Also, the normal alkaline phosphatase level makes bony injury less likely. Metastatic disease is also a possibility though again, the alkaline phosphatase would be expected to be high, the onset of the pain would probably be more gradual in most cases, and the plain radiographs are often, though not always, abnormal.

Osteomyelitis of the vertebral body can cause this type of pain and does not always cause the alkaline phosphatase to rise, so this is the closest differential diagnosis. Although an infected intevertebral disc is the most likely cause of the pain in this patient, it is essential to investigate promptly and thoroughly to confirm this, before starting treatment. The distinction from osteomyelitis is a fine one and, in many cases of septic discitis, there will be an adjacent osteomyelitis as a result of direct spread (**15**).

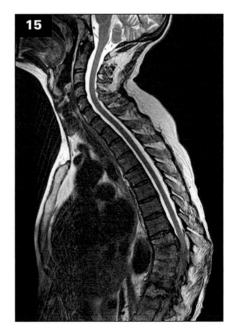

15 MR scan showing advanced discitis and associated bone involvement.

Tutorial (Patient 15)

Many cases of septic discitis are discovered at postmortem in patients who have died of unidentified sepsis. In recent years, probably due to better awareness and the availability of MR scanning, the diagnosis is more frequently made antemortem. The MR scan appearances are characteristic (15). Antibiotic treatment needs to be guided by bacteriological studies whenever possible to ensure an effective antibiotic regimen. Blood cultures will sometimes provide that information, though some patients may require direct sampling from the infected disc under imaging control if that is thought to be necessary in an individual case. In most patients the response to antibiotic treatment is excellent, with relatively early resolution of pain and the prospect of a return to full mobility.

Patient 16

A 90-year-old man was referred by the orthopaedic surgeons. He had been admitted, 10 days earlier, after he was knocked down by a car and was found to have fractured his left femoral neck. After operative fixation he developed pneumonia requiring ventilatory support in the intensive care unit for 2 days. He had previously been well for his age, able to walk slowly for more than 1 mile and was taking no medications before his accident. Now, he was unable to walk unaided due to weakness. He had no pain. On examination he was afebrile and had a MMSE score of 28/30. His pulse was 80 bpm and regular, heart sounds normal with no signs of heart failure. Examination of the chest, abdomen, CNS, and skin was normal. He had no significant joint disease other than the recent hip fracture. His quadriceps femoris muscles were wasted and he was not able to rise against gravity from a chair. On the MRC muscle power scale he scored 4/5 in all muscle groups.

Investigations (normal range)

Haemoglobin 11.9 g/dL (13–18)
MCV 89 fL (80–96)
Total white cell count 9.1 × 10^9/L (4–11)
Serum urea 3.1 mmol/L (2.5–7.5)
Serum sodium 139 mmol/L (137–144)
Serum potassium 3.4 mmol/L (3.5–4.9)
Serum albumin 29 g/L (37–49)
Serum total bilirubin 8 mmol/L (1–22)
Serum ALT 20 U/L (5–35)
Serum alkaline phosphatase 305 U/L (45–105)
Serum CK 74 U/L (24–195)
ESR 27 mm/h (<15)
ECG normal

1 The most important underlying reason for this patient's weakness is:
A Sarcopenia.
B Protein depletion.
C Hypokalaemia.
D Disuse atrophy.
E Anaemia.

2 The main histological change in skeletal muscle in old age is:
A Mitochondrial depletion.
B Reduced muscle fibre number.
C Inclusion body accumulation.
D Aberrant cell nuclei.
E Fatty infiltration.

3 The most effective treatment for age-related muscle weakness is:
A High protein diet.
B Potassium supplements.
C Muscle massage.
D Load-bearing exercise.
E Galvanic stimulation.

Patient 16 Answers

1 A Sarcopenia.

In a 90-year-old man the most likely background reason for his current generalized weakness is sarcopenia. By definition, sarcopenia is a reduction in muscle mass to less than two standard deviations below the mean for a young healthy reference group. Some reduction in muscle mass occurs universally with ageing and becomes particularly noticeable above the age of 80. In this patient the mild degree of hypokalaemia would not be enough, in itself, to explain his severe weakness, though it might be contributing and should be corrected. There is some evidence that the patient is truly protein-depleted in that he has a low serum albumin and has recently had a severe acute illness. However, although this might be making some contribution through exacerbating muscle wasting, it is not the principal cause in this case. For example, by comparison, a younger patient having suffered a similar illness and with the same serum albumin and potassium levels would not be expected to be too weak to rise from a chair. Some acute disuse atrophy could be contributing in this patient, though the illness was only of 10-days duration. From the patient's history, it would appear that he is normally sufficiently active to have prevented severe disuse atrophy over a prolonged time period. Patients who are bed-bound and chair-bound would fall into that category. The patient is not sufficiently anaemic to affect static muscle power.

2 B Reduced muscle fibre number.

Sarcopenic muscle in old age is characterized by a reduced number of muscle fibres. There is also a decrease in the diameter of those fibres (**16**). There is some evidence that mitochondrial dysfunction contributes to the sarcopenic state in old age, though there is no significant amount of mitochondrial depletion. Mitochondrial density in skeletal muscle is an important determinant of aerobic endurance but is not the principal factor in determining strength. Some inclusion bodies accumulate with age in virtually all nondividing cells, including myocytes. However, this is not thought to be an important factor in determining strength. The nuclei of aged myocytes do not look fundamentally different from those in younger patients on light microscopy. Some fatty infiltration occurs with age as adipose tissue accumulates and lean body mass falls. However, this condition is not unique to old age and can be seen in younger obese patients.

3 D Load-bearing exercise.

There is a substantial body of evidence to show that exercise programmes are the most effective treatment for age-related muscle weakness. Despite sarcopenic change, aged muscle responds to exercise and the patient can benefit from improved strength and aerobic endurance. The form of exercise is relatively unimportant but aerobic moderate load-bearing exercise such walking, cycling, and swimming are the most suitable for older people. Isometric exercises and high load-bearing exercises are also effective but in older patients those approaches are limited by adverse effects on joints and ligamentous structures. Galvanic stimulation can cause muscle contraction but it is not a proven or practical means to improve functional muscle strength. Massage can improve the sense of well-being and can reduce muscle tension but makes no contribution to improving muscle strength. Patients who are protein-depleted and potassium-depleted should receive supplementary protein and potassium in their diet and there will be some long-term benefit for the patient's general nutrition and muscle strength. However, these will not be effective on their own and are no substitute for a well-managed exercise programme.

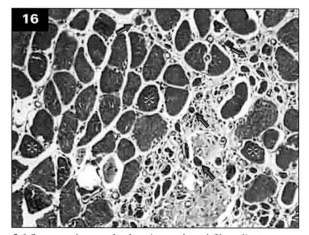

16 Sarcopenic muscle showing reduced fibre diameter (arrows) and normal fibres (stars).

Tutorial (Patient 16)

The pathogenesis of sarcopenia is not fully understood. There are changes in the number and density of motor neurone units supplying skeletal muscle, particularly in the lower limbs. There are also changes in the rate of neurotransmission in motor neurone axons. It is thought that these subtle denervation effects could contribute to the phenomenon of sarcopenia, possibly by analogy with the severe wasting that is seen in patients with motor neurone disease. The reason for the loss of muscle fibres and reduction in mean muscle fibre diameter is not known. Muscle fibres exhibit a reduction in peak attainable force when adjusted for fibre size and loss of fibre shortening velocity with ageing after the age of approximately 50 years.

Patient 17

An 81-year-old patient was admitted after a collapse. He had a BP of 80/50 mmHg and was complaining of severe abdominal pain. The chest radiograph on admission is shown (**17**).

1 What abnormality would most likely explain this patient's presentation?
   A Chilaiditi syndrome.
   B Cardiomegaly.
   C Pneumoperitoneum.
   D Consolidation.
   E Pneumothorax.

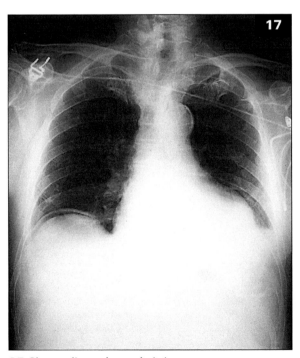

17 Chest radiograph on admission.

Patient 17 Answer

> **1 C** Pneumoperitoneum.

This patient has a pneumoperitoneum. There is a crescent of air visible under the right hemidiaphragm. Although there is cardiomegaly and possibly some consolidation or pleural thickening on the left, these would not explain the patient's presentation. This is a surgical emergency and is due to visceral perforation in 85–95% of cases. It can also be iatrogenically induced during laparoscopic surgery and may be present following a laparotomy.

An important differential diagnosis is the Chilaiditi syndrome. Intestinal hepatodiaphragmatic interposition is a rare condition recognizable by chest radiography (usually bowel haustrations are seen, unlike a pneumoperitoneum) and is most often asymptomatic. When symptomatic, the interposition may present with a variety of clinical symptoms and signs, mainly GI, but also with chest pain and dyspnoea. Certain groups are predisposed to this condition (elderly persons with constipation, the intellectually disabled, patients with chronic lung disease, emphysema, cirrhosis, and pregnant women). In elderly patients the differential diagnosis of chest pain and respiratory distress should include Chilaiditi syndrome among other GI disorders. The treatment is usually conservative (bed rest, increased fluid and fibre intake, laxatives, enemas), although rarely surgical intervention is needed, usually if there is a volvulus or obstruction.

Table 17a *Causes of abdominal pain in elderly patients*

• Idiopathic	• Duodenal ulcer
• Constipation	• Abdominal aortic
• Cholelithiasis	aneurysm
• Acute cholecystitis	• Appendicitis
• Intestinal obstruction	• Mesenteric ischaemia
• Acute pancreatitis	• Obstructive uropathy
• Gastroenteritis	• Volvulus
• Diverticulitis	

Tutorial

Acute abdominal pain is a common mode of presentation among elderly patients. At least 50% require hospitalization, 30–40% require surgery, and there is a mortality of around 10%. Elderly patients present differently compared with their younger counterparts. The elderly subjects have a high incidence of previously asymptomatic but potentially troublesome underlying pathology. Approximately one half of elderly patients have underlying cholelithiasis, one half have diverticular disease, and 5–10% have an AAA. Elderly patients often have underlying cardiovascular and pulmonary disease, which decreases cardio-respiratory reserve and predisposes them to conditions such as AAA and mesenteric ischaemia.

Elderly patients are more likely than younger patients to present with vague symptoms and have nonspecific findings on examination. Many have impaired cognitive function, allowing pathology to advance to a dangerous point prior to symptom reporting. An acute peritonitis in an aged person is much less likely to have the classic findings of an acute abdomen. They are less likely to have fever or leukocytosis. In addition, the pain can be much less severe than expected for a particular disease. This increases the risk that elderly patients with serious pathology are initially misdiagnosed as having benign conditions such as constipation or gastroenteritis.

Tables 17a, 17b provide a template to aid the differential diagnosis and examination of patients with abdominal pain.

Table 17b *Common anatomical pain sites of presentation for specific causes of acute abdominal disorders in elderly people*

Right hypochondrium and flank

• Cholecystitis	• Intestinal obstruction
• Pyelonephritis	• Retrocaecal appendicitis
• Penetrating ulcer	• Pancreatitis
• Choledocholithiasis	• Gastric ulcer

Epigastrium

• Pancreatitis	• Gastritis
• Duodenal ulcer	• Early appendicitis
• Penetrating ulcer	• Mesenteric ischaemia
• Colon carcinoma	• Abdominal aortic
	aneurysm

Left hypochondrium and flank

• Splenic enlargement	• Diverticulitis
• Pyelonephritis	• Bowel obstruction

Right iliac fossa

• Appendicitis	• Bowel obstruction
• Hernia	• Pyelonephritis
• Cholecystitis	• Diverticulitis
• Psoas abscess	• Leaking aneurysm

Hypogastrium

• Diverticulitis	• Cystitis
• Bladder obstruction	• Appendicitis
• Prostatism	• Hernia
• Bowel obstruction	• Colon carcinoma

Left iliac fossa

• Diverticulitis	• Bowel obstruction
• Hernia	• Leaking aneurysm
• Pyelonephritis	• Abdominal wall
	haematoma

Patient 18

An 85-year-old bed-bound woman with a long history of constipation presented acutely with vomiting, abdominal pain, and distension. A plain abdominal radiograph was obtained (**18**).

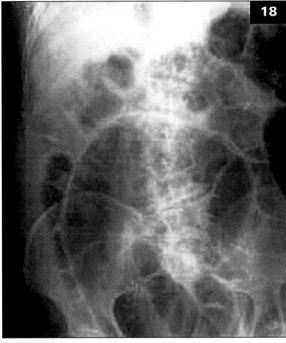

1 What would be the best initial intervention?
A Senna.
B Laparatomy.
C Flatus tube.
D Nasogastric tube.
E Hot water bottle.

18 Plain abdominal radiograph taken on admission.

Patient 19

A 78-year-old woman presented with a 3-month history of dyspepsia, anorexia, and significant weight loss. Physical examination revealed a BMI of 17 kg/m^2. She refused endoscopy but agreed to have a 'barium' meal performed (**19**).

1 What best describes the abnormality shown in the investigation below?
A Hiatus hernia.
B Linitis plastica.
C Gastric ulceration.
D Gastro-oesophageal reflux.
E Gastric cancer.

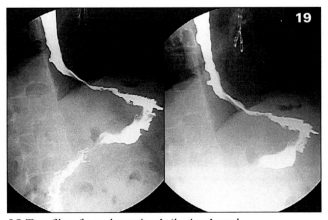

19 Two films from the patient's 'barium' meal.

Patient 18 Answer

1 C Flatus tube.

The abdominal radiograph reveals gross distension of the sigmoid and descending colon. The acute onset of the symptoms suggests volvulus as the diagnosis. The best initial intervention for this condition would be the insertion of a flatus tube under sigmoidoscopic guidance. With a history of constipation, now complicated by volvulus, it is unlikely that senna will be of any benefit. A laparotomy may be required at a later stage if the patient is fit for surgery. The condition can settle after insertion of a flatus tube so a laparotomy would not be a first line intervention. Apart from failed decompression, indications for urgent laparotomy are fever and leucocytosis that persist after decompression, and other clinical indications suggestive of intestinal ischaemia, perforation, or peritonitis. A nasogastric tube would give some symptom relief but would not deal with the volvulus and therefore is not the best answer. A hot water bottle is of no use in managing this condition.

Tutorial

Volvulus of the colon most commonly arises in the sigmoid colon followed by caecum, splenic flexure, and transverse colon. Sigmoid volvulus has variable geographical and racial distribution. It is extremely common in developing countries where it affects young male patients but has a lower incidence in the West where it affects mostly old and frail female patients. The aetiology of the condition remains speculative. While chronic constipation is blamed for the Western type of sigmoid volvulus, a high fibre diet has been deemed a major factor in the development of sigmoid volvulus in the African population. Sigmoid volvulus is produced when a long redundant sigmoid twists about its mesenteric axis in either direction and forms a closed loop obstruction. The degree of torsion is 360° in 50% of cases, 180° in 35% of cases, and 540° in 10% of cases.

The management of sigmoid volvulus involves relief of obstruction and the prevention of recurrent attacks. As with any colonic obstruction, bowel ischaemia and perforation can occur if prompt decompression is not achieved. Fluoroscopic or sigmoidoscopic guidance of a tube is successful in 70–90% of cases and therapeutic if vascular compromise is not severe. A rectal tube should subsequently be placed *in situ*. Sigmoidoscopic decompression carries the risk of perforation, particularly if there is a gangrenous intestine. Clinical signs of gangrene at sigmoidoscopy include a devitalized mucosa after reduction and bloodstained effluent from the sigmoidoscope or rectal tube. Where gangrene is suspected decompression should not be attempted before surgery. A barium enema examination may lead to reduction of a volvulus in 5% of patients. There is spontaneous resolution in 2% of cases. Sigmoid volvulus has a high recurrence rate of up to 80%. Recurrence is an indication for resection of the redundant sigmoid if the patient is fit for surgery.

Patient 19 Answer

1 B Linitis plastica.

The 'barium' meal shows marked constriction of the stomach cavity. The appearance is characteristic of linitis plastica also known as Brinton's disease. This is a diffuse infiltrative adenocarcinoma of the stomach.

Tutorial

This is a rare form of stomach cancer and the appearance of the stomach is often described as similar to a leather bottle. As the radiograph shows (**19**), there is often extensive mucosal erosion and coarse thickening of the gastric wall. The differential diagnosis of such a radiographic appearance would be lye ingestion and metastatic infiltration of the stomach. It differs from the most common form of stomach adenocarcinoma, which often presents as an ulcer. Linitis plastica spreads to the muscles of the stomach wall and makes it thicker and rigid. This means that the stomach has a reduced capacity and does not stretch or move as it should when food is ingested. This type of carcinoma has a very poor prognosis. It is more common in Asian countries, particularly Japan.

Patient 20

An 88-year-old woman who had been resident in a nursing home since a stroke 3 years ago, was found one morning to be a little more drowsy than usual and less able to communicate. She was dependent on nursing staff for all activities of daily living and had a long-term urinary catheter. The nurses suspected a UTI and a dipstick urinalysis was positive for protein, blood, nitrites, and leukocytes. On examination the patient was afebrile and had no abdominal tenderness. Her pulse, BP, and respiratory rate had not changed. A catheter specimen of urine was sent to the laboratory for microbiological analysis and her GP prescribed a 7-day course of amoxicillin. One week later she developed severe diarrhoea and mild lower abdominal pain. She had a temperature of 38.2°C, and her BP fell to 90/50 mmHg. No other residents or staff at the nursing home had diarrhoea. After further review by her GP, she was admitted to hospital.

The appearance of her sigmoid colonic mucosa is shown in Figure **20**.

1 Which of the following is the most likely cause of the diarrhoea?
 A Ischaemic colitis.
 B Nonspecific antibiotic-associated diarrhoea.
 C *Clostridium difficile* enterocolitis.
 D Norovirus infection.
 E *Salmonella* enteritis.

2 How firm was the evidence of UTI in this case?

3 What percentage of female nursing home patients without a urinary catheter will have a positive MSSU analysis (a positive test being defined as >100,000 bacteria and >10 leukocytes per high powered field)?

4 Which of the following courses of action would have been best when this patient was observed to be slightly more drowsy than usual at the beginning of the episode described above?
 A Prescribe trimethoprim rather than amoxicillin.
 B Wait for the result of the catheter specimen of urine and give antibiotics if it is positive.
 C Daily bladder irrigations with an antibacterial solution.
 D Continue to take observations and monitor the patient's clinical state.
 E Change the urinary catheter.

Investigations (normal range)

Haemoglobin 14.0g/dL (11.5–16.5)
Total white cell count 18.1×10^9/L (4–11)
Neutrophil count 17.0×10^9/L (1.5–7)
Serum urea 22.1 mmol/L (2.5–7.5)
Serum creatinine 120 µmol/L (60–110)
Serum sodium 151 mmol/L (137–144)
Serum potassium 3.6 mmol/L (3.5–4.9)
Serum albumin 38 g/L (37–49)
Serum total bilirubin 8 µmol/L (1–22)
Serum ALT 34 U/L (4–35)
Serum AST 29 U/L (1–31)
Serum corrected calcium 2.3 mmol /L
 (2.2–2.6)
Serum phosphate 1.1 mmol/L (0.8–1.4)

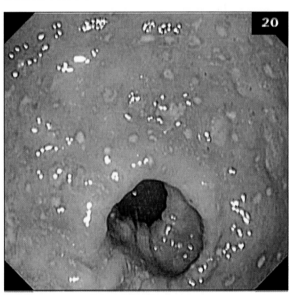

20 Appearance of sigmoid colonic mucosa.

Patient 20 Answers

> **1 C** *Clostridium difficile* enterocolitis.

> **4 D** Continue to take observations and monitor the patient's clinical state.

The best answer is *Clostridium difficile* enterocolitis. This diagnosis is suggested by the preceding course of antibiotics, the low-grade fever, and the relatively severe diarrhoea with lower abdominal discomfort. The diagnosis can be confirmed in most cases by the demonstration of *Clostridium difficile* toxin in the stool or by growth of the bacterium from a stool sample. Ischaemic colitis can cause diarrhoea but is usually associated with much more severe abdominal pain and blood staining of the diarrhoea. It is possible that this patient could have nonspecific antibiotic-associated diarrhoea, though that would be unlikely to cause a fever. Also, the diarrhoea is usually not as severe as that seen in the majority of cases of *Clostridium* enterocolitis. Norovirus infection can produce an illness such as that described in the case above, so it does remain in the differential diagnosis until laboratory evidence has confirmed the presence of *Clostridium difficile*. However, none of the other patients or staff in the nursing home had a similar illness, which makes an epidemic viral diarrhoea less likely. Similarly, *Salmonella* enteritis could cause the clinical picture described and needs to be included in the differential diagnosis. The lack of obvious exposure to a possible source of *Salmonella* and the lack of similar symptoms in other patients reduced the likelihood of salmonellosis in this case.

2 The diagnosis of UTI in this patient was made on weak evidence. The presence of protein, blood, nitrites, and leukocytes on routine urine analysis in frail elderly nursing home patients has a low specificity and sensitivity for significant UTI. Surveys have shown that between 30 and 60% of such patients will have a positive urinalysis, even if they have no symptoms. Therefore, urine testing of this type is more useful if it is found to be negative, in which case UTI is very unlikely. Furthermore, there were no dysuric symptoms in this patient. It is very important to avoid the temptation of using UTI as a catch-all pseudo-diagnosis to explain episodes of deterioration in frail elderly patients. Not only will this lead to patients being unnecessarily exposed to antibiotics, but it also reduces the likelihood of the correct diagnosis being pursued.

3 About 50% of frail elderly female nursing home patients without a urinary catheter will have a MSSU that shows >100,000 bacteria and >10 white cells per high power field. In similar patients with a long-term urinary catheter, that figure rises to more than 80%. Therefore, a positive MSSU or catheter specimen of urine also has a low sensitivity and specificity for detecting clinically significant UTI in elderly nursing home residents.

In the patient described, the best option was to continue to take observations and monitor the patient's clinical state. Frail elderly patients often fluctuate in their level of consciousness, particularly those with extensive cerebrovascular disease or dementia (the greatest fluctuations are associated with Lewy body dementia and related states). In many cases the apparent problem will resolve without recourse to extensive investigations and interventions. If any of the basic observations or physical signs changes, that would then prompt a possible need for further action. Giving trimethoprim rather than amoxicillin might slightly reduce the risk of subsequent *Clostridium* enterocolitis, though there was really no indication to give any antibiotic to this patient. As described above, the value of a catheter specimen of urine without other evidence of UTI is not of much help, so giving antibiotics on the strength of that result alone would not be indicated. Bladder washouts are useful for removing solid materials suspended in urine (such as crystals or blood), and can help to avoid a blocked catheter. There is no firm evidence that bladder washouts, with or without antibacterial solutions, have any significant effect on the attack rate from genuine urinary tract sepsis. Similarly, there was no indication in this patient to change the urinary catheter under the circumstances described.

> ## Tutorial
>
> *Clostridium difficile* enterocolitis is an extremely important GI infection with a strong iatrogenic factor in its causation through the prescription of antibiotics. While there is no doubt that certain antibiotics carry a much higher risk of causing this complication, such as clindomycin and cephalosporins, it is also seen as a complication of more commonly used antibiotics such as amoxicillin and trimethoprim. Of course, antibiotics are life-saving when used appropriately; however, thoughtless over-use of antibiotics poses a substantial risk, particularly in frail older people, who have a high level of morbidity and a significant mortality from *Clostridium* enterocolitis.

Patient 21

A 79-year-old female, resident in a nursing home, was referred for assessment. She had an 8-year history of paraplegia caused by a spinal cord infarction at D6 level but had managed at home with a wheelchair, hoist, and visits from a care team three times daily. She fell from her bed when trying to transfer herself to the wheelchair, spent 9 hours on the floor and developed a large sacral pressure sore (21); this was the reason for her admission to the nursing home. About 5 weeks later the ulcer was clear of necrotic tissue but granulation tissue was growing slowly and patchily; the ulcer base appeared not to be healing. For 2 weeks her appetite had decreased and a low-grade pyrexia was observed that had not responded to a trial of trimethoprim for a suspected, but not proven, urinary tract infection. For 3 days immediately prior to her assessment hard granular material had been seen in the exudate from the base of the pressure sore and the patient reported worsening sacral pain. Her medication consisted of paracetamol 1 g 8 hourly and codeine phosphate 15 mg as required. The investigations below were carried out by her GP 2 days before the assessment.

Plasma protein electrophoresis showed a polyclonal rise in IgG but no monoclonal band. A catheter specimen of urine was positive on routine testing to blood, protein, nitrites, and leukocytes, and had a mixed growth of bacteria.

1 Which of the following investigations is most likely to provide the best diagnostic information?
A Wound swab for bacterial culture.
B Biopsy of the ulcer base for bacterial culture.
C Plain radiograph of the sacrum.
D Isotope bone scan.
E MR scan of the sacrum and pelvis.

2 At this stage, which of the following methods of ulcer treatment is the best option?
A Vacuum-assisted dressing.
B Peroxide-based dressing.
C Nonadherent deep wound dressing at atmospheric pressure.
D Occlusion dressing with larval debridement.
E Antibiotic-impregnated dressing.

3 Pressure sores are normally graded from 1 to 4. Define the grades.

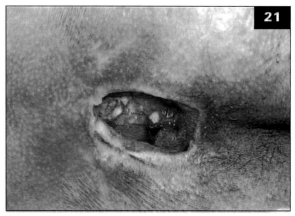

21 Pressure sore on the sacrum.

Investigations (normal range)

Haemoglobin 9.9 g/dL (11.5–16.5)
Total white cell count 17.2 × 10⁹/L (4–11)
Neutrophil count 15.8 × 10⁹/L (1.5–7)
Serum urea 9.0 mmol/L (2.5–7.5)
Serum creatinine 84 µmol/L (60–110)
Serum sodium 144 mmol/L (137–144)
Serum potassium 4.4 mmol/L (3.5–4.9)
Serum ALT 17 U/L (5–35)
Serum alkaline phosphatase 382 U/L (45–105)
Serum total bilirubin 13 µmol/L (1–22)
Serum albumin 28 g/L (37–49)
Serum corrected calcium 2.4 mmol/L (2.2–2.6)
ESR 74 mm/h (<30)
Serum CRP 122 mg/L (<10)

Patient 21 Answers

| 1 E MR scan of the sacrum and pelvis. | 2 C Nonadherent deep wound dressing at atmospheric pressure. |

The best option is an MR scan of the sacrum and pelvis. The patient has several clinical features to suggest osteomyelitis in the underlying sacral bones; these include the low-grade pyrexia, neutrophil leukocytosis, high ESR and CRP, polyclonal rise in IgG, delayed healing of the pressure sore, and the presence of granular material at the ulcer base (indicative of bone destruction). A wound swab in such circumstances will always grow a variety of organisms. The relationship between such a swab and uncontrolled infection adjacent to the ulcer is not clearcut. If osteomyelitis is suspected, a culture might be useful if it grows a specific organism such as MRSA, though cause and effect cannot be assumed. The same applies for a biopsy of the ulcer base as this will also be populated by a wide range of bacteria, even in a healthy ulcer that is healing normally. Plain radiographs of the sacrum might reveal osteomyelitis if it is advanced. In this patient there might be some changes, since there are other clinical features of bone destruction. However, plain radiographs are unlikely to indicate the extent of the osteomyelitis and could miss it altogether. An isotope bone scan is likely to be abnormal but provides nothing like the anatomical detail that is obtained by performing an MR scan. Furthermore, MR scanning can also provide information about collections of pus and inflammation in nonbony tissue adjacent to the sacrum.

At this stage a nonadherent deep wound dressing at atmospheric pressure would be best. Vacuum-assisted dressings are known to speed up ulcer healing once debridement has taken place and granulation tissue is beginning to form. However, in the presence of proven or suspected osteomyelitis or other deep infection, the method is contraindicated. Peroxide-based dressings are no longer used as they suppress the growth of granulation tissue. Occlusion with larval debridement is useful when necrotic tissue is proving difficult to remove. That was not the problem in the case described above, as general debridement was satisfactory. It would also not be standard practice to use larval debridement in the presence of suspected underlying bone infection. In the case described, there is no indication for an antibiotic-impregnated dressing. Once osteomyelitis was confirmed by MR scanning, systemic antibiotics were required.

3 There are several systems of classification for pressure sores. The most common classification, used extensively in the UK, is as follows:
- **Grade 1** – an area of erythema without necrosis or ulceration.

Tutorial

Pressure sores form when blood flow to tissue ceases due to sustained pressure. The critical factor is pressure that exceeds mean capillary perfusion pressure, which is around 25 mmHg in patients with a normal systemic BP. Damage occurs to skin and muscle if blood flow is not restored within around 2 hours, so patients with insufficient mobility to redistribute their body weight are at high risk. On a foam mattress a patient lying supine will have pressures of around 60–70 mmHg over the sacrum, 30–45 mmHg over the heels, and around 40 mmHg at the occiput and scapulae. Shearing forces can also obstruct capillary blood flow, as can folding of loose tissue. The key factor in pressure sore avoidance is to maintain blood flow through vulnerable areas by using techniques such as regular turning, special pressure distribution beds, for example large-cell ripple mattresses, and correct positioning of the patient and bed clothes to avoid shearing and folding. Other important risk factors are outlined in *Table 21*.

Table 21 *Risk factors for pressure sores*

- Any condition that causes severe limitation of mobility, such as stroke, Parkinson's disease, spinal cord injuries
- Any condition leading to a severe reduction in the level of consciousness, but particularly coma
- Conditions causing a reduction in cardiac output or blood pressure, for example cardiogenic shock, septicaemia, GI haemorrhage
- Severe underlying arteriosclerotic disease to the extent that mean capillary perfusion pressure in the peripheries is reduced
- Any cause of hyperviscosity; this drastically reduces flow in capillaries compromised by pressure
- Severe, uncontrolled metabolic conditions such as diabetic ketoacidosis, probably through reduction in the efficiency of peripheral utilization of oxygen
- Sedative or analgesic drugs that reduce the patient's instinct to move around spontaneously, or reduce or remove pain and discomfort from areas of high pressure

- **Grade 2** – ulceration of the skin with little necrosis of subcutaneous tissues and no involvement of underlying muscles or other structures.
- **Grade 3** – a deeper ulcer with necrosis of deep structures including muscle.

- **Grade 4** – a very severe ulcer with exposure of deep structures such as bone and tendons, and the formation of extensive undermining cavities.

Patient 22

An 80-year-old man was referred to clinic with increasingly frequent falls and deteriorating memory. His family reported that he was well until 2 months earlier. His previous medical history consisted of a prostatectomy for benign prostatic hypertrophy 10 years ago, gastroesophageal reflux disease, and hypertension. His medication was bendroflumethiazide 2.5 mg daily and omeprazole 20 mg at night. Systems review revealed no other important information. On examination he was afebrile. He found it difficult to concentrate and was easily distracted. His AMTS was 5/10, MMSE 16/30, and FAB 3/14 (normal >8). His pulse was 84 bpm and regular, heart sounds normal, BP 145/85 mmHg. His JVP was normal. Respiratory rate was 14 per minute and auscultation of his lung bases was normal. There were no abnormalities found on examination of the abdomen or the skeleto-muscular system. CNS examination revealed no definite abnormal cranial nerve signs. Power and sensation were normal and there was no clear cerebellar ataxia. However, he was clumsy, bilaterally dyspraxic, and had very poor balance. His deep tendon reflexes were rather brisk but symmetrical with flexor plantar reflexes and no primitive reflexes. During the examination three myoclonic jerks were observed involving the face and arms.

A routine specimen of urine was negative for blood protein, nitrites, and leukocytes. His chest radiograph was reported as normal and he had a normal ECG. A CT head scan showed mild cerebral atrophy but was otherwise normal. An EEG had the appearances shown in Figure **22a**.

Investigations (normal range)

Full blood count, serum urea, creatinine and electrolytes, screening liver function tests and thyroid function all normal
ESR 25 mm/h (<20),
Serum corrected calcium 2.3 mmol/L (2.2–2.6)

Lumbar puncture showed:
Opening pressure of 170 mm of water (50–180)
CSF total protein 0.60 g/L (0.15–0.45)
CSF glucose 3.9 mmol/L (3.3–4.4)
CSF total white cell count 7/μL (<5)
CSF lymphocyte count 70% (60–70)
No organisms seen on Gram staining and no growth on culture

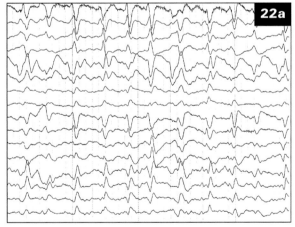

22a EEG taken soon after initial assessment.

1 Which of the following is the most likely diagnosis?
  A Herpes simplex encephalitis.
  B NPH.
  C Drug-induced encephalopathy.
  D Complex partial seizures.
  E CJD.

2 A firm diagnosis in this case would best be achieved by:
  A MR brain scan.
  B PET scan of the brain.
  C Brain tissue histology.
  D Assay for neuronal protein 14-3-3 in CSF.
  E Serological analysis of blood for antibodies against slow viruses.

Patient 22 Answers

1 E CJD.	**2 D** Assay for neuronal protein 14-3-3 in CSF.

The most likely cause of this man's neurological presentation is CJD. This is supported by the subacute onset, the mixed cognitive and motor signs, the myoclonic jerks, and the EEG abnormality. Herpes simplex encephalitis is usually a much more acute illness and there are usually more definite CSF abnormalities. NPH can certainly present with a cognitive deficit and gait disorder, though it would not normally be associated with myoclonic jerks; the CT head scan would be abnormal, showing a disproportionate enlargement of the brain ventricles in comparison with relatively compressed sulcae. A drug side-effect is always a possibility, though the drugs in this patient's case are not normally associated with encephalopathy. Furthermore, the EEG appearance is supportive of the diagnosis of CJD in this case. The progressive nature of the neurological abnormality in this man effectively rules out complex partial seizures as in such cases the clinical picture would be expected to be intermittent unless there was complex partial status epilepticus, in which case the patient would usually be expected to have presented more acutely.

An absolutely firm diagnosis in suspected CJD can only be made by the examination of brain tissue. This is usually done at postmortem and is very rarely done while the patient is still alive. Strongly supportive evidence for CJD can be obtained by analysis of the CSF for the neuronal protein 14-3-3, though this is not specific for CJD and can be raised in other inflammatory brain disorders, such as viral encephalitides. MR brain scanning can be normal in CJD, though nonspecific abnormalities in the midbrain have been reported in advanced cases. Some patients with new variant CJD have a characteristic MR abnormality known as the Pulvinar sign (**22b**). There is no diagnostic yield from PET scanning in suspected CJD, and blood serological tests for the condition have not been developed.

Tutorial

If a patient is suspected of having CJD, it is important to rule out the differential diagnoses, such as low-grade viral encephalitis and infiltrating malignant disorders such as gliomatosis cerebri. Patients who have a neurological condition progressing over a number of months, with progressive cognitive impairment, motor disorders (commonly first manifested as a severe balance disorder), and myoclonic jerks are likely to be suffering from CJD, particularly if they also have a normal CT brain scan, typical abnormalities on the EEG, and the presence of neuronal protein 14-3-3 in CSF. Patients with all of these features will usually prove to have CJD when their brain tissue is examined at postmortem. It is important to try to establish the diagnosis so that the patient and his/her family can be given some idea of the likely course of the disease and a proper plan can be made for palliative care. Patients with suspected or probable CJD should be referred to the appropriate specialist department so that material can be sampled for disease confirmation and, in the case of possible new variant CJD, disease prevalence monitoring and tracking for possible exposure through blood transfusion.

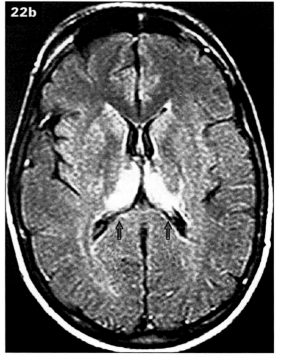

22b Pulvinar sign on MR in new variant C CJD.

Patient 23

A 79-year-old man who normally lived independently was brought to the hospital by his son who had found him crawling on the floor of his house after falling. He had been incontinent of urine and was disorientated in time and place. He was a smoker with a 50 pack-year exposure and had had a diagnosis of COPD made by his GP, after spirometry, 2 years earlier. His only medication was aminophylline modified release 225 mg twice daily. Examination revealed a tympanic membrane temperature of 37.6°C, pulse 90 bpm irregularly irregular, BP 140/85 mmHg, respiratory rate 28 per minute with reduced expansion and use of accessory muscles of respiration. Auscultation of the chest revealed inspiratory and expiratory rhonchi and coarse crackles at both lung bases; all the chest signs were symmetrical. There was loss of liver and cardiac dullness. CNS examination showed no obvious lateralizing neurological signs but was difficult to perform as the patient was anxious and uncooperative.

An ECG showed atrial fibrillation (this was not present on his previous ECG) and right bundle branch block (this was not new). A chest radiograph was taken and is shown (**23a**). Spirometry performed by his GP 3 months earlier showed a reduction of the FEV1 to 40% of predicted and FVC to 65% of predicted, and little response to inhaled salbutamol. Visual assessment of sputum showed a tinge of yellow with no blood and a very sticky consistency. A diagnosis of acute exacerbation of COPD was made.

Investigations (normal range)

Haemoglobin 18.4 g/dL (13–18)
Haematocrit 0.56 (0.4–0.52)
Total white cell count 10.2×10^9/L (4–11)
Neutrophil count 9.2×10^9/L (1.5–7)
Serum urea 6.1 mmol/L (2.5–7.5)
Serum sodium 139 mmol/L (137–144)
Serum potassium 4.8 mmol/L (3.5–4.9)
Serum ALT 24 U/L (5–35)
Serum total bilirubin 9 mmol/L (1–22)
Serum alkaline phosphatase 390 U/L (45–105)
   (alkaline phosphatase values between 350
   and 400 had been noted for the last 4 years)
Arterial blood gas estimation breathing air
   showed:
pH 7.4 (7.36–7.44)
PO_2 6.8 kPa (11.3–12.6)
PCO_2 7.1 kPa (4.7–6)
Bicarbonate 22 mmol/L (19–24)
Oxygen saturation 86%

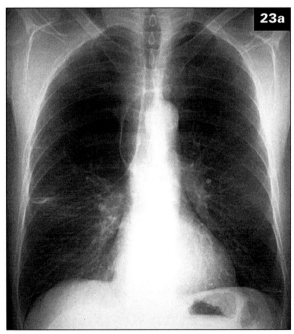

23a Chest radiograph taken on admission.

1 In addition to nebulized bronchodilators and oral corticosteroids, the treatment most likely to resolve the presenting problems is:
   A Digoxin.
   B Aminophylline.
   C Intravenous fluids.
   D Oxygen.
   E Antibiotics.

2 The most important prophylactic treatment for this patient at the acute stage is:
   A Clexane.
   B Tamcyclovir.
   C Pneumococcal vaccine.
   D Omeprazole.
   E Risedronate.

3 Which of the following is the most likely reason for the patient's raised alkaline phosphatase level?
   A Primary hyperparathyroidism.
   B Paget's disease of bone.
   C Osteomalacia.
   D Bony metastases.
   E Multiple myeloma.

Patient 23 Answers

---

1 D Oxygen.

The patient presented with disorientation and incontinence and was substantially hypoxic breathing room air. It is likely that these presenting symptoms are largely due to hypoxic cerebral dysfunction, though there may be a contribution from the low-grade fever. The patient is mildly hypercapnic so caution needs to be exercised with the oxygen concentration. In this case it would be reasonable to start with 24% and not rise above 28% oxygen. Blood gas monitoring is mandatory under these circumstances and the patient's condition should be tracked using a properly designed oxygen prescription chart. With these precautions, if there is a worsening of the patient's hypercapnoea, appropriate further assessment can take place to decide whether the patient should have any form of assisted ventilation.

There is no urgent need for digoxin since the atrial fibrillation is not associated with an unacceptably high ventricular rate. Further aminophylline should not be given intravenously unless the patient's blood aminophylline levels are known and, in any case, there is not likely to be a dramatic response to aminophylline in this context. The patient does not have evidence of dehydration on biochemical analysis and it is likely that the high haemoglobin and haematocrit are due to long-term hypoxia (secondary polycythaemia) rather then haemoconcentration. Therefore, fluids should be offered orally and only given intravenously if absolutely necessary. Although it is probable that this patient's exacerbation has been precipitated by infection, there is no good evidence of overwhelming bacterial infection and it is more likely to be due to a virus such as respiratory syncytial virus. Many patients are given antibiotics under these circumstances though in this patient's case it would be hard to justify. Certainly, it is more important to give oxygen supplementation.

---

2 A Clexane.

The patient has new-onset atrial fibrillation and is hypoxic, and is therefore at a substantial risk of thromboembolic disease. That risk can be reduced with prophylactic doses of subcutaneous low-molecular weight heparin. There is no indication to give tamcyclovir in this man. He might benefit from pneumococcal vaccination in the autumn as a long-term prophylactic strategy, though there would be no reason to give it during this acute illness. Omeprazole prophylaxis is not indicated under these clinical circumstances. If he requires long-term systemic corticosteroid therapy or frequent recurrent short-term corticosteroid treatments, it would be sensible to give risedronate to provide osteoporosis prophylaxis. This does not need to be done as part of his acute management.

---

3 B Paget's disease of bone.

The patient is known to have had a high but stable alkaline phosphatase level for several years. The most common cause of that observation in older people is Paget's disease of bone. A radiograph of his hip is shown (**23b**). Primary hyperparathyroidism would be expected to cause a high corrected calcium which this patient does not have. Osteomalacia causes a rise in alkaline phosphatase but would be associated in most cases with a low corrected calcium and symptoms of osteomalacia such as bone pain, myalgia, and proximal muscle weakness. Bony metastases will also cause a rise in alkaline phosphatase, though this would be expected to be progressive rather than stable over several years and the patient would be expected to have other symptoms and signs of disseminated malignancy. The same applies to multiple myeloma, which in this man's case is unlikely because of the lack of bone pain, normal calcium, and absence of anaemia or renal dysfunction.

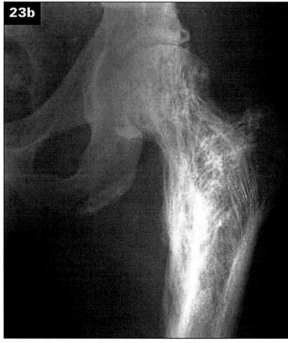

23b Radiograph of the left hip showing changes caused by Paget's disease (deformity, trabecular disorganization, areas of lysis, and sclerosis).

Tutorial (Patient 23)

Elderly patients presenting with acute exacerbations of COPD require prompt assessment and treatment. Attention needs to be paid to the correction of hypoxia and careful fluid balance. Patients benefit from bronchodilator therapy, usually with a combination of a beta-agonist and antimuscarinic agent, and from suppression of airways inflammation with corticosteroids. Unless there are contraindications, patients fulfilling the criteria for supported ventilation should be offered that treatment promptly, supervised in an appropriate environment such as a high dependency unit or acute lung unit. Proper assessment and management of co-morbidities is essential and thromboembolic prophylaxis for the immobile hypoxic patient is crucial.

Antibacterial treatments should be given if there is a strong suspicion of bacterial infection (new inflammatory infiltrate on chest radiograph, definite neutrophil leukocytosis, sustained high body temperature, positive blood cultures, or extremely purulent and copious sputum). Patients with probable noninfective or viral exacerbations should not be given antibiotics because of the risk of antibiotic associated diarrhoea and the generation of resistant organisms.

Patient 24

An 88-year-old man was brought to the Rapid Access Geriatric Clinic by his daughter. For about 10 days he had become lethargic, increasingly drowsy, and intermittently confused. Two falls had occurred, each within a few seconds of rising from a chair. He had a history of peripheral vascular disease, angina, and hypertension. He had a 50 pack-year smoking history, but stopped smoking about 8 years ago. His medication was bendroflumethiazide 2.5 mg daily, diltiazem slow-release 120 mg daily, isosorbide mononitrate 10 mg twice daily, lisinopril 10 mg daily (started 4 weeks earlier because of poor control of his hypertension), quinine sulphate 200 mg daily, aspirin 75 mg daily, and simvastatin 20 mg daily. On examination his body temperature was 36.8° C and he was disorientated in time and place, with a GCS of 14/15, pulse 66 bpm and regular, normal heart sounds, JVP raised 4 cm, and BP 135/75 mmHg. His respiratory rate was 22 per minute and there were very scanty medium crackles at both lung bases. Examination of the abdomen and skeleto-muscular system was normal. His feet were cool and no foot pulses were palpable, though femoral pulses were present on both sides. There were no focal neurological signs.

Basic liver function screen was normal. An ECG showed nonspecific T-wave flattening and T-wave inversion in the lateral leads. A chest radiograph showed a cardiothoracic ratio of 50% and slight hyperinflation but was otherwise normal. Routine specimen of urine was positive for protein but was otherwise normal. Blood taken by the patient's GP 6 weeks earlier had shown a urea of 11.2 mmol/L and creatinine of 105 μmol/L.

Investigations (normal range)

Haemoglobin 12.4 g/dL (13–18)
Total white cell count 8.2×10^9/L (4–11)
Neutrophil count 7.2×10^9/L (1.5–7)
ESR 29 mm/h (<20)
Serum urea 55.2 mmol/L (2.5–7.5)
Serum creatinine 550 μmol/L (60–110)
Serum sodium 138 mmol/L (137–144)
Serum potassium 5.9 mmol/L (3.5–4.9)
Arterial blood gases breathing air showed:
PO_2 of 9.9 kPa (11.3–12.6)
PCO_2 4.1 kPa (4.7–6.0)
pH 7.37 (7.36–7.44)
Bicarbonate 14 mmol/L (19–24)

1 The most likely cause of this man's renal failure is:
   A Abdominal aortic dissection.
   B Dehydration.
   C End-stage renovascular disease.
   D Renal arteriosclerosis.
   E Renal vein thrombosis.

2 The most important next step in the patient's management is:
   A Insertion of a central venous pressure line.
   B Stop the lisinopril.
   C Intravenous colloid infusion.
   D Haemofiltration.
   E Acute peritoneal dialysis.

3 Which of the following tests is most likely to explain the falls:
   A Gait analysis.
   B Tilt Table Test.
   C Measurement of lying and standing BP.
   D 24-hr ECG recording.
   E CT head scan.

Patient 24 Answers

1 D Renal arteriosclerosis.

The most likely reason was renal arteriosclerosis. The patient was known to have had only slightly impaired renal function 6 weeks before presentation and had had an ACE-I (lisinopril) started 4 weeks earlier. In patients with stenosed renal arteries there is frequently an abrupt deterioration in renal function when an ACE-I is added to their treatment regimen. Abdominal aortic dissection is usually more catastrophic than the clinical picture in this case, and it is more likely that the patient will present anuric if the renal arteries have been involved in the dissection. Also, there would not have been time for the metabolic acidosis to have adequately compensated as was the case in this patient. There were no features strongly suggestive of dehydration, either in the history or the biochemical results, though once patients become drowsy or confused an inadequate fluid intake often exacerbates their renal dysfunction. The patient is unlikely to have end-stage renovascular disease because the renal function was almost normal only 6 weeks earlier. Renal vein thrombosis is a relatively rare condition and tends to present more acutely than in this case. The likelihood of this patient having bilaterally narrowed renal arteries due to arteriosclerosis is further reinforced by his age, smoking history, hypertension, and peripheral vascular disease.

2 B Stop the lisinopril.

It is important to stop the lisinopril. In a patient in whom there has been an abrupt deterioration in renal function after starting an ACE-I, there is a strong likelihood that renal function will improve quickly after stopping the drug. In patients with renovascular disease, ACE-Is reduce renal plasma flow and glomerular filtration rate much more dramatically than they do in people with relatively normal renal arteries. Of course, patients with hypertension, mild to moderate renovascular disease, and diabetes are known to benefit from long-term treatment with ACE-Is, providing they can take them without a major and sustained deterioration in renal function.

There is no indication for a central venous pressure line in this patient since he is haemodynamically stable and not acidotic. Central venous lines have their own associated hazards, including sepsis, and should only be inserted when absolutely necessary. The patient is unlikely to benefit from a colloid infusion since there is every reason to think his circulating blood volume is adequate (normal BP and slightly raised JVP). This indicates that there is unlikely to be any significant

prerenal component to this patient's renal failure. Haemofiltration as an urgent procedure is not indicated in this patient since he is not dangerously hyperkalaemic or acidotic. Furthermore, there is every reason to expect his renal function to improve on stopping the ACE-I. Acute peritoneal dialysis is now very rarely performed in modern health systems.

3 C Measurement of lying and standing BP.

The description of the falls, occurring shortly after rising from a chair, suggests that the patient has orthostatic hypotension. This will best be detected by measuring his BP in the lying and standing positions. He also has other risk factors for postural hypotension, including several antihypertensive drugs and a long-acting nitrate preparation. Although the gait of any patient with falls should be assessed, the history in this case does not suggest a primary gait disorder. Tilt Table testing of this patient would almost certainly reveal the orthostatic hypotension but that investigation should not be used solely for that purpose. There are no features to suggest that the patient has a significant rhythm disorder and no indications in this case to perform a CT head scan.

Tutorial

Before starting treatment with an ACE-I or angiotensin II receptor blocker, a baseline serum creatinine value should be measured. The serum creatinine should be remeasured a few days after starting the treatment. A small rise in creatinine will occur in a large proportion of patients. As a rule of thumb, if this rise is <30% and then reaches a new steady state, treatment should be continued, and there is evidence that there will be a long-term beneficial effect on renal function. Somewhat larger rises in creatinine can be acceptable in individual patients, particularly when an ACE-I is resulting in improved control of breathlessness in a patient with left ventricular failure. However, if there is a relentless rise in the creatinine, the drug will have to be stopped or, as in this case, a severe degree of renal failure can occur and the patient's metabolic homeostasis can be compromised.

Patient 25

An 81-year-old woman telephoned her GP to report that she was unable to walk because of extreme pain in her right foot that came on while she was asleep. The GP visited and found severe tenderness across the plantar aspect of the foot so asked a geriatrician to see the patient at her home. She felt otherwise well, and was normally able to walk unaided. Her previous medical history consisted of a hysterectomy for menorrhagia 45 years earlier, a possible TIA 3 years ago, type 2 diabetes mellitus controlled by diet, and hypertension recently diagnosed at a Well Elderly Screening Clinic. Her medication consisted of bendroflumethiazide 2.5 mg daily, atorvastatin 10 mg daily and aspirin 75 mg daily. By the time the domiciliary visit was carried out 4 days later, the foot was almost pain-free but the patient's left 5th finger had become swollen and painful (**25**). On examination she was afebrile and looked well. She weighed 58 kg and her body mass index was in the normal range. Her Abbreviated Mental Test Score was 9/10. Her pulse rate was 78 bpm and regular, BP 135/90 mmHg, respiratory rate 12 per minute, and no abnormalities were found on auscultation of the heart or chest. Examination of the abdomen and CNS was normal and the only abnormalities on examination of the skeleto-muscular system were extreme tenderness over the proximal interphalangeal joint of the left 5th finger, and some residual tenderness on pressure at the centre of the plantar surface of the right foot. She was a non-smoker and her alcohol intake was consistently less than 10 units/week.

An ECG showed sinus rhythm and slightly high voltages over the left ventricular leads but was otherwise normal.

---

1 List the differential diagnosis in order of likelihood.

2 Which of the following blood tests is most likely to help clarify the diagnosis?
  A Rheumatoid factor.
  B Autoimmune profile.
  C Serum uric acid.
  D Serum phosphate.
  E Serum CRP.

3 Which is the most likely cause of the foot pain?
  A Trauma.   **D** HLA B27-related
  B Gout.   enthesitis.
  C Pseudo-gout.   **E** Infection.

4 Comment on the patient's drug history in the context of this clinical presentation.

5 The most likely reason for her raised serum ALT level is:
  A Diabetic hepatosteatosis.
  B Aspirin toxicity.
  C Metastatic disease of the liver.
  D Biliary tract disease.
  E Atorvastatin therapy.

Investigations (normal range)

Haemoglobin 13.7 g/dL (13–18)
MCV 90 fL (80–96)
Total white cell count 5.7 × 10⁹/L (4–11)
Neutrophil count 5.0 × 10⁹/L (1.5–7)
ESR 20 mm/h (<20)
Serum urea 8.4 mmol/L (2.5–7.5)
Serum creatinine 100 µmol/L (60–110)
Serum sodium 141 mmol/L (137–144)
Serum potassium 3.7 mmol/L (3.5–4.9)
Serum albumin 42 g/L (37–49)
Serum total bilirubin 4µmol/L (1–22)
Serum ALT 55 U/L (5–35)
Serum alkaline phosphatase 71 U/L (45–105)
Serum corrected calcium 2.5 mmol/L (2.2–2.6)

25 Painful left 5th finger.

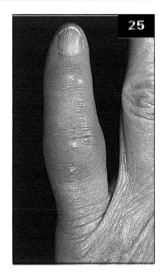

Patient 25 Answers

1 The patient has had the acute onset of pain at two sites, one a joint and one a soft tissue compartment with no other symptoms of ill health. There is also no history of trauma. Therefore, it is most likely that the patient has a noninfective inflammatory condition and in conjunction with that, it is unlikely that there is a serious systemic inflammatory disorder. Consequently, the most prominent potential diagnosis is gout with crystal deposition in the ligamentous structures of the sole of the foot and in the 5th proximal interphalangeal joint on the right. Sepsis is a possibility, though unlikely, and other rheumatological conditions with an autoimmune basis need to be included in the differential diagnosis but are also very unlikely. Such conditions would include rheumatoid disease, SLE, sero-negative arthropathies and post-infective arthropathies. The clinical context in this case makes all of those differential diagnoses very unlikely. Elderly patients with gout often present in the typical manner with involvement of the 1st or 2nd metatarsophalangeal joints. However, with increasing age, there is a trend towards atypical presentation including other joints such as the fingers, knees, or ankles and soft tissue structures such as the plantar fascia, tendon insertions, and entheses.

---

2 C Serum uric acid.

As the most likely diagnosis is gout, immediate support for that diagnosis would be gained by demonstrating a raised serum uric acid level. Of course, a proportion of patients with gout will have a normal serum uric acid level and there is a tendency for the serum urate to fall slightly during an active attack of gout. However, the majority of patients with gout will have an abnormally raised serum uric acid. Rheumatoid factor is unlikely to help in this patient's case as the clinical presentation is not typical of rheumatoid disease, and it is unlikely that an autoimmune profile would be helpful as there is no evidence of a more generalized autoimmune process or specific autoimmune disease. It also has to be remembered that a substantial proportion of elderly patients will have one or more autoantibodies present without any manifestation of autoimmune disease. There is no indication for measuring the serum phosphate in this patient and in patients with pseudo-gout, the serum phosphate would be normal. The CRP level might be slightly high in patients with an acute attack of gout but that would also be true of the majority of acute inflammatory arthropathies so it would not help to resolve the diagnosis. Of course, a very high CRP level would not be consistent with gout (though can be high in pseudo-gout) and would indicate the need for further investigation.

---

3 B Gout.

The most likely cause of the foot pain is gouty plantar fasciitis. This is supported by the clinical presentation and the patient's otherwise good health. Trauma is unlikely in this patient since she is compos mentis and gives no history of trauma. Furthermore, the pain came on while the patient was asleep which would be unusual if the cause was trauma. Pseudo-gout tends to involve larger joints such as the knees and wrists, though it can cause an acute monarthropathy in a digit. However, pseudo-gout is confined to joints and does not cause crystal-induced inflammation in other structures such as ligaments and the plantar fascia. HLA B27-related enthesitis is a feature of ankylosing spondylitis and is a recognized cause of plantar surface foot pain. However, the clinical context, with the involvement of a hand joint, points away from this. Furthermore, it tends to be a more chronic condition with a peak incidence in younger people. Infection is unlikely as there were no physical signs of infection, and the patient was afebrile with a normal white cell count and ESR.

4 The patient had recently been diagnosed as having hypertension and was taking bendroflumethiazide. It can therefore be deduced that she was started on the bendroflumethiazide relatively recently. Thiazide diuretics are a risk factor for gout as they reduce the renal clearance of uric cid. Furthermore, low-dose aspirin also reduces renal excretion of uric acid so the two drugs combined can predispose a patient to overt gout. Consequently, the drug history in this patient is also strong supporting evidence for the diagnosis of gout.

---

5 E Atorvastatin therapy.

Statins often cause a small stable rise in liver transaminase levels in serum. This is not an indication to stop treatment unless it is progressive. Some sources also recommend stopping treatment if the level rises higher than four times the upper limit of normal. Fatty infiltration of the liver (hepatostatosis) is associated with a rise in ALT, usually in patients with abdominal or visceral obesity, but is less likely in this patient as she is slim. Metastatic disease usually causes a more diffuse range of liver function test abnormalities. Biliary obstruction would initially cause a rise in the serum bilirubin and alkaline phosphatase levels. Low-dose aspirin rarely causes abnormalities of liver function.

Tutorial (Patient 25)

Gout is a common condition in old age that can present with the full spectrum from acute gout, as in the case described, through to chronic tophaceous gout and chronic gouty arthritis. It is important to make the diagnosis because the acute phase responds extremely well to NSAIDs and, for patients with persistent or recurrent gout, longer term management by suppressing uric acid synthesis with allopurinol can help older patients to avoid episodes of immobility and distressing pain. Generally speaking, gout should be investigated and treated in older people along the same lines as for people in middle age. Sufferers should be advised to avoid excess alcohol intake, reduce weight if they are obese, avoid foods with a high purine content, and keep themselves well hydrated. Drugs that reduce uric acid secretion should be avoided if possible. Other conditions often associated with gout such as hypertension and hyperlipidaemia should be optimized. For frail older patients with marginal mobility in whom walking is compromised by, for example, an acutely gouty knee, it is justifiable to gain rapid control of the arthropathy with an intra-articular injection of corticosteroid, once the diagnosis has been confirmed by the demonstration of uric acid crystals in the joint aspirate.

Patient 26

A 90-year-old man was brought to the Accident and Emergency Department by his niece. She had visited him for the first time in 5 weeks and found him disorientated and talking about seeing objects on the walls of his flat. He was not perturbed by any of this and thought she was making too much fuss. On direct questioning he described intermittent visual hallucinations consisting of bright lines and complex patterns against the walls or carpets, with no particular time pattern or obvious precipitating events. He did admit that his vision had become much worse in the last 2 months. He had a medical history of a Duke's A carcinoma of the sigmoid colon, resected 8 months previously, hypertension, pernicious anaemia, and senile macular degeneration. He spontaneously acknowledged that the visions he had been seeing were not real and he understood them to be aberrations of vision. On examination he was afebrile with a MMSE score of 27/30. His visual acuity was clearly very poor, being reduced to 6/60 on the right and light/dark discrimination on the left. On examination of his optic fundi the degenerative changes associated with macular degeneration were clearly seen but the appearances were otherwise normal. His pulse was 86 bpm and regular, BP 135/80 mmHg lying, 128/80 mmHg standing. Examination of his chest and abdomen were normal apart from the scar from his previous surgery. His skeleto-muscular system was in good condition for a man of his age and there were no focal neurological signs. His balance was normal and he was able to walk safely with the aid of a stick. He had smoked about 5 cigarettes/day for most of his adult life. His drugs consisted of amlodipine 10 mg daily and vitamin B12 injections 3-monthly.

A chest radiograph was reported as normal, routine dipstick testing of urine was negative, and his ECG showed no significant abnormalities. Reports from his visual acuity testing 18 months previously confirmed a loss of central vision with overall acuity of 6/60 on the right and 6/30 on the left.

Investigations (normal range)

Haemoglobin 13.6g/dL (13–18)
MCV 93 fL (80–96)
Total white cell count 5.5×10^9/L (4–11)
Neutrophil count 4.7×10^9/L (1.5–7)
ESR 17 mm/h (<20)
Serum urea 7.4 mmol/L (2.5–7.5)
Serum sodium 139 mmol/L (37–144)
Serum potassium 3.8 mmol/L (3.5–4.9)

---

1 The most likely cause of this man's hallucinations is:
 A Schizophrenia.
 B Drug toxicity.
 C B12 deficiency amblyopia.
 D Lewy body disease.
 E Visual sensory deprivation.

---

2 Which of the following tests would be the most useful next investigation:
 A Visual field charting.
 B CT head scan.
 C MR scan of the orbits.
 D Measurement of anterior chamber pressure.
 E Occipital cortex PET scan.

---

3 What is Bonnet's syndrome?

Patient 26 Answers

---

1 E Visual sensory deprivation.

2 D Measurement of anterior chamber pressure.

The most likely reason for this man's visual hallucinations is visual sensory deprivation. This is supported by the fact that he now has very poor vision, he is otherwise in good health, and he retains good insight into the abnormality of his visual aberrations. Schizophrenia rarely causes visual hallucinations; auditory hallucinations are far more common in that condition; furthermore, in a truly psychotic illness the patient would have other psychotic features and would not retain insight. Acute psychotic illnesses can occur for the first time in old age, but it would be very unusual for them to present with isolated visual hallucinations. Drug toxicity is a possibility though the patient's current drug regimen is not one that is normally associated with abnormalities of vision. If drug toxicity causes delirium, or the drugs have a direct hallucinogenic effect, the patient normally presents in a more agitated state and there may be other psychological or psychiatric features. B12 deficiency amblyopia is unlikely to have caused the recent deterioration in this man's vision since he has been on vitamin B12 replacement therapy. Blindness as a result of vitamin B12 deficiency is extremely uncommon and the majority of patients with vitamin B12 deficiency present with other features of that condition before blindness occurs. Heavy smoking in conjunction with vitamin B12 deficiency is associated with accelerated tobacco amblyopia but that condition is also uncommon and is very unlikely in this case. The hallucinations of Lewy body disease can have the characteristics of those described in this patient. However, the patient has none of the other characteristics of Lewy body disease so that makes option D less likely. Figure 26 shows an example of senile macular degeneration.

The history suggests that the patient's vision has deteriorated rapidly in the last few weeks, so is unlikely to be due to progression of the underlying senile macular degeneration as that is a gradual process over many years. Therefore, a possible second cause for impaired vision should be sought in this man. In an elderly person, one of the most treatable conditions would be glaucoma, so the best next test would be to measure the anterior chamber pressure to confirm or rule out that condition. Visual field charting would be useful in this man to assess the deterioration in vision from the senile macular degeneration and the possible superimposed effects of glaucoma, though that would not need to be done urgently. A CT head scan is unlikely to contribute much in this man's case as he has no other neurological symptoms or signs; however, visual hallucinations can be an early symptom of visual cortex diseases, including neoplasms, so a CT scan could be justified as part of the overall investigation plan for the patient. An MR scan of the orbits is unlikely to contribute in this patient and there is nothing to be gained from conducting a functional PET scan of the occipital cortex.

3 Bonnet's syndrome consists of very clear and complex visual hallucinations depicting scenery, individuals, or animals occurring in patients with severe bilateral visual impairment. It appears to be independent of the underlying cause of the blindness. Patients find the images nonthreatening, though they may seek medical advice as to the significance of the hallucinations. Patients living alone appear to be more prone to developing Bonnet's syndrome in the context of visual sensory deprivation. It is likely that Bonnet's syndrome is simply an extreme form of the colour and shape hallucinations described in the patient above. The mechanism of Bonnet's syndrome hallucinations is not known, though it is thought that the lack of normal visual stimuli releases complex visual scenes from memory.

26 Senile macular degeneration.

Patient 27

An 86-year-old woman fell from a top step and hit her head on a concrete patio. This injury was witnessed. She was rendered unconscious and was taken to hospital by ambulance. Her GP was able to provide information by telephone that she suffered from ischaemic heart disease with stable angina, hypertension, and type 2 diabetes mellitus. She had had a mastectomy for carcinoma of the breast 2 years ago with no evidence of metastatic disease at the last review. On examination she had a GCS of 8/15, core body temperature of 34.6°C and a laceration of her skull in the left postero-lateral position. Her pulse was 90 bpm irregularly irregular, BP 180/100 mmHg with no signs of cardiac failure. Her respiratory rate was 14 per minute and there were no abnormalities on auscultation of her chest. Her pattern of breathing was regular. She had normal pupillary reflexes and no focal neurological signs were found. Her GCS score did not rise over the next 2 hours. It was found that her medications consisted of slow-release diltiazem 120 mg/day, aspirin 75 mg/day and gliclazide 60 mg/day. Investigations were performed immediately after her admission.

An ECG showed atrial fibrillation with a rate of about 95 per minute with T-wave inversion over the inferior leads, but no signs of acute coronary insufficiency and no diagnostic features of MI. A chest radiograph showed no significant abnormalities and a skull radiograph showed no evidence of a fracture. Oxygen saturation on room air was 96%.

Investigations (normal range)

Haemoglobin 11.3 g/dL (11.5–16.5)
MCV 88 fL (80–96)
Total white cell count 10.3 × 10⁹/L (4-11)
ESR 24 mm/h (<30)
Serum urea 10.1 mmol/L (2.5–7.5)
Serum creatinine 110 mmol/L (60–110)
Serum sodium 140 mmol/L (137-144)
Serum potassium 4.4 mmol/L (3.5–4.9)
Random plasma glucose 16.4 mmol/L (3–8.5)

1 The factor most closely associated with a poor prognosis in this patient is:
   A Her age.
   B Her core body temperature.
   C The blood glucose level.
   D The GCS score.
   E The presence of atrial fibrillation.

2 The most useful next investigation is:
   A Cardiac enzyme assay.
   B CT head scan.
   C Lumbar puncture.
   D EEG.
   E Measurement of HbA1C.

3 The most important immediate management priority is:
   A Rewarming.
   B Lower the blood sugar.
   C Airway maintenance.
   D Further investigation.
   E Reduction in the systemic BP.

4 If the CT head scan shows no significant abnormality, the most likely cause of this patient's unconsciousness is:
   A Concussion.
   B Hypothermia.
   C Dehydration.
   D Diabetic ketoacidosis.
   E Sepsis.

Patient 27 Answers

---

1 D The GCS score.

There is a strong association between a GCS score of 8 or less and high mortality in elderly patients after head injury. The same applies to a reduced GCS due to other conditions in old age. The only condition with a stronger association is persistent severe hypotension not responding to treatment. In older patients head injury does carry a poor prognosis but age in itself is not the most powerful predictive factor. In this patient the body temperature was only slightly in the hypothermic range at 34.6°C, which is not associated with a poor outcome. A blood glucose level of about 16 mmol/L in itself would not be a major predictor of a poor outcome in this patient, though diabetic patients often have substantial co-morbidities related to diabetic vascular disease that can contribute to a poorer outcome. Atrial fibrillation with a ventricular response of around 90 bpm is of little prognostic value. A new onset of atrial fibrillation sometimes signifies underlying serious acute conditions such as myocardial infarction, pulmonary embolism, or sepsis, though there was no evidence in this case to support any of those diagnoses.

---

2 B CT head scan.

In the context of a severe head injury, it is essential to rule out potentially treatable intracranial trauma, even when there are no firm neurological signs other than the reduced level of consciousness. Therefore, it would be sensible to proceed immediately to a CT head scan, particularly to detect any intracranial haemorrhage. The cardiac enzymes might be raised in such a patient if there has been an associated MI, though total creatine kinase would not be very useful as there would almost certainly be skeletal muscle injury from a severe fall. There is no indication for lumbar puncture in this case and no reason to perform an EEG. The HbA1C level would give some overall idea of the patient's diabetic control in the medium term but need not be performed as an urgent investigation.

---

3 C Airway maintenance.

Patients with a GCS score of 8 or less are extremely vulnerable to aspiration of pharyngeal or refluxed gastric contents into their airways. Therefore, airway maintenance is the most important immediate priority. Patients with this level of GCS associated with an absent gag reflex should be considered for endotracheal intubation. The patient does not require active rewarming; it is likely that her body temperature will rise to the normal range naturally once she is indoors and under blankets. It would certainly be necessary to recheck the temperature after an hour or so to make sure that the core body temperature has not fallen further. There is no urgent need to lower the blood sugar, though it should be monitored and appropriate action taken if it continues to rise. Some type 2 diabetic patients in these circumstances might need insulin to control their blood sugar during the acute illness. While the investigations are important, they should wait until the patient has a secure airway. The patient's level of hypertension is not dangerously high; so, in this clinical scene, the most appropriate option would be to continue to measure the BP as one of the regular observations on an unconscious patient. A steadily rising BP in these circumstances can be an indication of rising intracranial pressure.

---

4 A Concussion.

After a head injury, if the CT scan shows no evidence of intracranial bleeding or other acute pathology, it is most likely that the patient is simply concussed. Elderly patients are more prone to concussion than younger adults. Also, the recovery phase from a concussion often takes longer in old age. The patient is not sufficiently hypothermic to cause unconsciousness and there is no reason to suspect from the history that she is dehydrated. The slightly high urea and creatinine are likely to be a consequence of her diabetic and hypertensive state. Although it would be possible for her to have diabetic ketoacidosis with a blood sugar of 16.4 mmol/L, that would be unusual and the patient was not observed to have an increased respiratory rate and tidal volume, as might be expected in a metabolic acidosis. However, it would be prudent to perform a blood gas estimation on this patient as a means of assessing her acid–base status. There is no evidence of infection in this case, though sepsis should be considered as part of the differential diagnosis of a patient with a reduced GCS of uncertain cause.

Tutorial (Patient 27)

Head injuries are common in older people, largely due to the higher prevalence of falls in patients with postural instability. Head injuries are a marker of frailty and there is a strong association between head injury and dependent outcomes. In old age the dura mater becomes firmly adherent to the skull, so extradural haematomas are rarely seen in elderly patients with head injury. However, cerebral atrophy due to ageing or dementia leads to increased fragility in the veins bridging the subdural space, thereby increasing the risk of subdural haematomas. Consequently, some patients develop subdural haematomas after very minor head trauma and those patients characteristically show a fall in GCS score after presentation to hospital. Some patients benefit from neurosurgical evacuation of intracranial haematomas. Outcomes are better in patients with good preinjury functional scores, fewer co-morbidities, absence of dementia, and good renal function.

Patient 28

A 75-year-old woman complained of sleepless nights. She mentioned an urgent desire to move her legs due to intolerable tingling. Often, she had to get out of bed to obtain symptom relief. Physical examination was normal.

1 What is the most likely primary cause of her presentation?
   A Painful peripheral neuropathy.
   B Restless legs syndrome.
   C Peripheral vascular disease.
   D Guillain-Barré syndrome.
   E Iron deficiency.

Investigations (normal range)

Haemoglobin 8.5g/dL (11.5–16.5)
Total white cell count 4.5 × 10⁹/L (4–11)
Platelet count 350 × 10⁹/L (150–400)
MCV 70 fL (80–96)
Serum iron binding capacity 90 µmol/L (45–75) TIBC
Screening blood tests of renal, liver and thyroid function normal
Random plasma glucose 4.2 mmol/L

Patient 29

An 85-year-old patient known to have advanced dementia was admitted urgently after a fall. He politely declined to be seen by the consultant on the posttake ward round. The patient claimed that he had no time to chat as he was waiting for the bus to be taken to school and had been told by his mother not to speak to strangers.

1 What would be the best course of action?
   A Orientate and divert him.
   B Give haloperidol and come back later.
   C Ignore him and move on to the next patient.
   D Contradict the patient.
   E Ask him where is the bus stop.

Patient 28 Answer

1 E Iron deficiency.

This woman has symptoms suggesting the restless legs syndrome. A distinction needs to be made between idiopathic restless legs syndrome, which is the commonest form, and secondary restless legs, which is due to an underlying condition such as iron deficiency anaemia or renal failure. As this woman has a low haemoglobin with a low MCV and a raised TIBC, she has an iron deficiency state and that is the most likely cause of her presentation.

Tutorial

Restless legs syndrome is also known as Ekbom's syndrome after the Swedish neurologist who first described it in the 1940s. It is characterized by sensory symptoms and a motor disturbance of the limbs, mainly during rest.

Four basic elements must be present to make the diagnosis:
- A desire to move the limbs, often associated with paraesthesia or dysaesthesia.
- Symptoms exacerbated by rest and relieved by activity.
- Motor restlessness.
- Nocturnal worsening of symptoms.

In most cases, restless legs syndrome is idiopathic. Such idiopathic disease can be familial (in 25–75% of cases) and, if so, is transmitted in an autosomal dominant pattern. Before attributing restless legs to idiopathic disease, secondary causes need to be excluded. A list of possible causes is given in *Table 28*.

The most effective drugs to treat the condition are dopaminergic agents such as L-dopa, ropinorole or cabergoline. Also useful are clonazepam, opioids, gabapentin, and clonidine. Additional agents are available that may be beneficial as add-on or alternative therapy.

Table 28 *Factors and conditions that may contribute to secondary restless legs syndrome (in approximate order of frequency)*
- Iron, folate, or magnesium deficiency
- Polyneuropathy (alcohol abuse, amyloidosis, diabetes mellitus, idiopathic polyneuropathy, lumbosacral radiculopathy, Lyme disease, MGUS, RA, Sjögrens's syndrome, uraemia, vitamin B12 deficiency)
- Pregnancy
- Anaemia
- Parkinson's disease
- Gastric surgery
- COPD
- Carcinoma
- Chronic venous insufficiency or varicose veins
- Intake of certain substances or drugs, e.g. alcohol, caffeine
- Medications such as anticonvulsants (e.g. phenytoin), antidepressants (e.g. amitriptyline, paroxetine), beta-blockers, histamine 2 antagonists, lithium, neuroleptics
- Withdrawal from vasodilators, sedatives, or imipramine
- Cigarette smoking
- Myelopathy or myelitis
- Hypothyroidism or hyperthyroidism
- Acute intermittent porphyria
- Fibromyalgia

Patient 29 Answer

1 A Orientate and divert him.

Orientate and divert is the best answer. This is a common experience when dealing with dementia patients. Attempting to orientate the patient, for example by telling him that he is in hospital, and diverting the subject by talking about something else, is the best way to try to establish trust with the patient. Giving haloperidol in this case is totally unwarranted and may paradoxically increase this patient's confusion. Ignoring or contraindicating the patient can lead to anger and a deterioration in the patient's behaviour. Asking where is the bus stop is likely to confirm the patient's false belief and, if the patient has periods of lucid thought, he might become suspicious of such a statement.

Patient 30

An 87-year-old woman was brought to hospital when her niece telephoned for an ambulance because she was so worried about her aunt's rapid deterioration in a nursing home. The nursing home staff were reluctant to seek help. On arrival the patient was confused and drowsy. She had been admitted to the nursing home after a series of falls and because of moderate dementia. She had been unable to walk for about 1 year. On examination she was in night clothes. Her AMTS was 0/10 and GCS 12/15. She was afebrile with a pulse of 90 bpm regular, BP 165/95 mmHg, and respiratory rate of 16 per minute. Examination of her chest and abdomen was otherwise normal. CNS examination was difficult but her right plantar reflex was extensor. There was a transverse deep ulcer on the posterior aspect of her right thigh just below the right buttock (**30a**). Both her thumbs were bruised (**30b**), but no other injury was found. Her GCS continued to fall so a CT head scan was performed (**30c**). A chest radiograph, ECG, and basic haematology and biochemistry tests were normal.

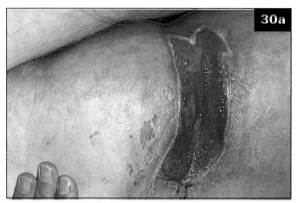

30a An unusual ulcer on the posterior aspect of the right thigh.

1 The CT head scan shows:
  A Extradural haematoma.
  B Cortical infarction.
  C Meningioma.
  D Subdural haematoma.
  E Intracortical haemorrhage.

2 How long has the intracranial pathology been present?

3 How might the leg ulcer and the thumb bruises be related?

4 The most likely mechanism for the leg ulcer in this patient is:
  A Self harm.
  B Pressure necrosis.
  C Arterial insufficiency.
  D Pyoderma gangrenosum.
  E Electrical burning.

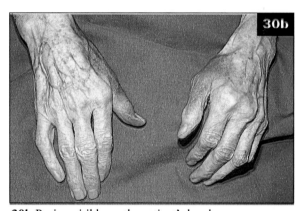

30b Bruises visible on the patient's hands.

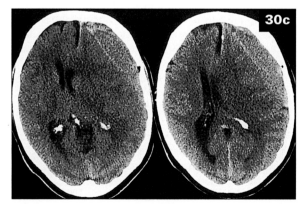

30c Two CT head scan slices taken due to the patient's deteriorating level of consciousness.

Patient 30 Answers

1 **D** Subdural haematoma.

The CT scan shows the typical appearances of a subdural haematoma. Extradural haematomas are uncommon in elderly patients and usually have more circumscribed edges (**30d**). A cortical infarction would be within the brain itself, whereas the lesion depicted shows displacement of the brain by the haematoma. Meningiomas are relatively radiodense and characteristically have a tail due to spread along the meninges. Intracortical haemorrhages would show as a relatively radio-opaque signal within the brain cortex.

2 The subdural haematoma shown in Figure **30c** is approximately isodense with the adjacent brain tissue. This indicates that it has been present for about 7–14 days. Subdural haematomas of more recent onset are more radiodense due to the presence of fresh blood. As the blood is gradually absorbed, the radiodensity falls, passing through an isodense phase until it becomes relatively radiolucent after approximately 2 weeks. A chronic subdural haematoma therefore, has low radiodensity, though fresh recurrent bleeding into a subdural haematoma can cause a mixed appearance, as can settling of blood cells under the influence of gravity.

3 The bruises on the thumbs in this patient are characteristic of those caused by an attendant pulling the patient up from a chair holding the thumbs in a reverse handgrip. In some cases this can be simply due to lack of skill, though it is also an indicator of possible physical abuse. The presence of an unusual skin lesion, the bruised thumbs, and the reluctance of the nursing home staff to seek help prior to the admission to hospital should alert the attending physicians to the possibility of unskilled, inappropriate, or overtly abusive handling of an elderly person. In such a case, the residential or nursing home in question should be referred to the appropriate licensing authorities so that an inspection or enquiries can be made. Clinicians seeing these types of injuries should always obtain photographs and detailed descriptions, and record them in the patient's clinical notes. Social services should also be informed in case there is a need to include the patient on an adult 'at risk' register.

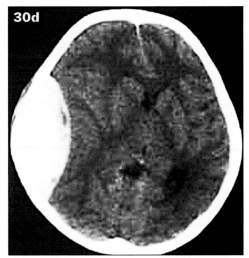

30d CT head scan showing an extradural haematoma.

4 **B** Pressure necrosis.

The unusual tranverse deep ulcer on the patient's leg is most likely to be due to pressure necrosis in this case. In fact, in the patient in question, it was caused by the patient having been left sitting on a commode for almost 4 hours with the consequent formation of a tranverse pressure sore at the point at which the patient's buttock was against the rim of a portable toilet. A close scrutiny of Figure **30a** will show that the wound had already been debrided and some epithelial healing had started at the wound edges. Deliberate self harm is always a possibility, though uncommon in elderly patients with dementia. It is most unlikely in this patient because of the site of the injury and the deep wound. Arterial insufficiency is very unlikely to occur in the upper part of the thigh as there is an ample collateral blood supply. Arterial insufficiency ulcers are almost always seen below the knee. The appearances are not those of pyoderma gangrenosum as there is no florid imflammatory ragged edge to the ulcer. An electrical burn is a possibility, though there was no history to support that and the adjacent skin showed no evidence of electrical damage.

Patient 31

A 75-year-old man was referred to the outpatient clinic. His wife had insisted on his being referred by the GP because her sleep had been disturbed for almost 2 years by her husband's increasingly frequent episodes of thrashing about and calling out in his sleep. These episodes were now occurring on most nights. On several occasions she had been bruised by blows from her husband's legs and had started to become distressed and even frightened of sleeping with him. She described him as being asleep during the attacks, though she was able to wake him with difficulty. He often remembered vivid dreams and reported these to his wife after being woken during an episode. He had no other complaints and felt completely well. He was taking no medication and had no significant previous medical history. On examination he looked well and was of strong build. Pulse was 66 bpm and regular, heart sounds normal, BP 130/85 mmHg. Examination of his chest and abdomen was normal. Detailed CNS examination was entirely normal. He had one bruise on his forehead from hitting his head on the bedside table during an attack.

Basic investigations, performed by his GP were entirely normal including a full blood count, urea, sodium and potassium, thyroid function, chest radiograph, and ECG. His ESR was 14 mm/h (<20). His wife, acting on advice from an Internet site, arranged for him to have an EEG performed privately (**31**).

1 The most likely diagnosis is:
   A Nocturnal epilepsy.
   B Restless legs syndrome.
   C Nocturnal hypoglycaemia.
   D REM sleep behaviour disorder.
   E Hypnogogic myoclonus.

2 In this particular patient, the best first line of treatment is a nightly dose of:
   A L-dopa.
   B Pramipexole.
   C Clonazepam.
   D Quetiapine.
   E Gabapentin.

3 What features should be looked for at follow-up?

4 What key investigations should be performed if neurological signs appear?

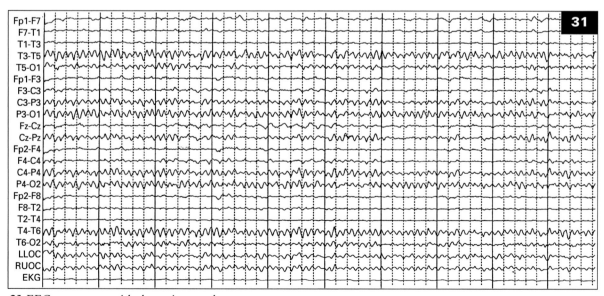

31 EEG appearance with the patient awake.

Patient 31 Answers

---
1 D REM sleep behaviour disorder.

The description of this patient's condition most closely fits the diagnosis of REM sleep behaviour disorder. This condition is characterized by violent movements of all limbs and vocalizations while the patient is dreaming during the REM phase of sleep. Nocturnal epilepsy is unlikely, partly because of the typical description of the REM sleep disorder and the fact that the patient can be wakened and reports that he is dreaming at the time. The absence of other features of generalized epilepsy such as incontinence and tongue-biting also reduce the likelihood of that diagnosis. The patient is not describing the classic features of restless legs syndrome. In that condition the patient complains that, while they are awake, they have an irresistible urge to move their legs to relieve the feelings of tension and unusual sensations in the lower limbs. The patient described in this case was always asleep when the abnormal movements took place. Nocturnal hypoglycaemia has to be considered in any patient with unusual neurological features coming on during fasting. It is usually seen in patients on treatments for diabetes mellitus, such as insulin and sulphonylureas, where hypoglycaemia is an unwanted feature and a sign of poor control. After waking, the patient had no other hypoglycaemic symptoms and had no risk factors for hypoglycaemia. Nevertheless, it would be prudent to check a night time blood sugar if there is any doubt about the diagnosis. Hypnogogic myoclonus is seen in patients of all ages and is a normal phenomenon that occurs in some individuals as they are initially drifting into sleep. The symptom is usually that of one or two muscular jerks and is sometimes associated with a sensation of falling. The patient usually wakes transiently and then returns to sleep.

---
2 C Clonazepam.

As the most likely diagnosis in this patient is REM sleep behaviour disorder, the first line treatment of choice is clonazepam. This is effective in the majority of patients with REM sleep behaviour disorder at a dose of 0.5 or 1 mg at night. In idiopathic cases (see below) clonazepam is virtually always successful. Some patients with REM sleep behaviour disorder associated with extrapyramidal disease such as Parkinson's disease, Lewy body disease, and progressive supranuclear palsy, will respond better to L-dopa or pramipexole. There is no evidence of benefit from tranquillisers such as quetiapine. There are individual case reports of benefit with a range of anticonvulsant drugs including gabapentin, though that should not be the first line of treatment.

3 The patient described had no neurological symptoms other than the presenting complaint and no abnormal neurological signs. However, REM sleep behaviour disorder is thought to be part of the Lewy body spectrum of conditions, so at follow-up it would be very important to look for subtle neurological deficits, particularly in the extrapyramidal system, and for evidence of dementia. Any signs of Parkinsonism, progressive supranuclear palsy, multi systems atrophy, or cognitive decline should prompt further investigation.

Tutorial

The prevalence of REM sleep behaviour disorder is not really known. Some studies have indicated that, in the general adult population, about 1 in 200 individuals would meet the criteria. Most of these do not have a severe or persistent form of the illness so relatively few patients present to medical services for help. Cases are usually described as idiopathic if there are no associated neurological symptoms and signs, and no abnormalities on brain imaging. The idiopathic pattern is generally seen in older people and is thought to be probably due to age-related degenerative changes or minor ischaemic change in midbrain and upper brainstem structures, though recent evidence suggests that Lewy body processes are the main underlying pathology. When the condition is secondary to other illnesses, the prognosis and mortality are determined by the pattern of the underlying disease. The condition is very rare under the age of 50, after which there is a steady and increasing frequency with age.

The most important associated conditions are brainstem neoplasms, Lewy body dementia, Alzheimer's disease, progressive supranuclear palsy, multi system atrophy, and multiple sclerosis. The incidence of the condition is higher in patients with Parkinson's disease and in all Parkinson's plus syndromes. Although the restless legs syndrome is a separate clinical entity, there is some overlap such that patients with REM sleep behaviour disorder have a higher prevalence of restless legs syndrome than the general population. This is probably due to the common involvement of dopaminergic systems in the pathophysiology of both conditions. Another closely related condition known as periodic limb movement during sleep needs to be differentiated, though this condition usually consists of very brief movements, lasting a few seconds, occurring every 30 seconds to a minute or thereabouts. It is more closely related to the restless legs syndrome and is less likely to respond to clonazepam.

4 If any neurological symptoms or signs are present at presentation, or if they emerge during follow-up, a CT or MR scan of the head should be performed. When lesions are present they are usually found in the upper brainstem and pons and tend to be fairly small, so there is probably a better yield from MR scanning. If there is doubt about the diagnosis, video-somnography should be performed, during which the patient has a video recording of their behaviour made during sleep. In the vast majority of cases this will confirm or refute the suspected diagnosis. An EEG is of limited value in such cases, and in this patient it was normal.

Patient 32

A 78-year-old woman was referred for an urgent outpatient review by her GP. She was complaining of increasing pain in her right hip. This was particularly severe on weight bearing and on flexion of the hip. There was a longer history, over about 18 months, of steadily worsening pain in the right hip. There was no history of recent falls but she had received operative treatment for a fracture of the right neck of femur 3 years previously after she fell from her bicycle. She was otherwise well and taking no long-term treatments. Recently, her GP had prescribed meloxicam 7.5 mg twice daily for the pain. On examination she was afebrile but clearly distressed by pain. Her AMTS was 9/10 and MMSE 27/30. Her pulse was 90 bpm and regular, BP 145/90 mmHg. Examination of the cardiovascular system, chest, abdomen, and CNS revealed no abnormalities. The left hip was normal. The right hip was limited to 20° flexion by pain and the right leg was shortened by approximately 3 cm. Her other joints were normal in the context of her age.

A chest radiograph was reported as normal and a radiograph of her right hip is shown in Figure **32**.

> *Investigations (normal range)*
>
> Haemoglobin 12.2 g/dL (11.5–16.5)
> Total white cell count 6.4 × 10⁹/L (4–11)
> ESR 18 mm/h (<30)
> Serum urea 7.9 mmol/L (2.5–7.5)
> Serum creatinine 83 mmol/L (60–110)
> Serum sodium 140 mmol/L (137–144)
> Serum potassium 3.6 mmol/L (3.5–4.9)
> Serum albumin 44 g/L (37–49)
> Serum corrected calcium 2.3 mmol/L (2.2–2.6)
> Serum phoshate 1.0 mmol/L (0.8–1.4)
> Serum total bilirubin 6 mmol/L (1–22)
> Serum alkaline phosphatase 83 U/L (45–105)
> Plasma free thyroxine 8 pmol/L (10–22)

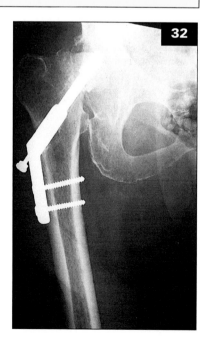

32 Radiograph of the painful right hip.

> **1** What does Figure **32** show?

> **2** In this patient the most important risk factor for the condition shown in the radiograph is:
> **A** Vasculitis.   **D** Trauma.
> **B** Hyperviscosity.   **E** Hypothyroidism.
> **C** The patient's age.

> **3** The most appropriate management for this condition in the patient described is:
> **A** Total hip replacement.
> **B** Hemiarthroplasty.
> **C** Girdlestone operation.
> **D** Anaesthetic hip block.
> **E** Replacement of the dynamic hip screw.

Patient 32 Answers

1 The radiograph shows evidence that a fractured hip has been repaired with a dynamic hip screw. However, avascular necrosis has taken place in the femoral head which is now distorted and in the process of being resorbed. Consequently, the tip of the dynamic hip screw is now eroding the surface of the acetabulum and that is the most likely source of the pain.

2 D Trauma.

In the patient described, the most important risk factor for avascular necrosis was the trauma to the hip at the time of hip fracture. Patients with intertrochanteric fractures usually have a preserved blood supply to the femoral head so the bone remains viable and can be repaired with a dynamic hip screw. In this patient it is likely that the blood supply was interrupted at the time of the trauma or was insufficient at a later stage to preserve bone integrity. There is no evidence of vasculitis in this patient, either clinically or on investigations (normal ESR, normal full blood count, and normal renal function). Similarly, patients with hyperviscosity would usually have a high ESR. Old age in itself is not a major risk factory for avascular necrosis of the femoral head. In fact, there is some evidence that the peak risk occurs in middle age when the fat cells within the bone marrow are large and tightly packed, which predisposes the bone to avascular necrosis. Although the patient in question had a low serum thyroxine level, this is not known to be a risk factor for avascular necrosis of the femoral head.

3 A Total hip replacement.

The best treatment for this condition, once there is associated damage to the acetabulum, is total hip replacement. This patient would probably not do well with a hemiarthroplasty, mainly because of the probable damage to the acetabulum by the tip of the dynamic hip screw. The Girdlestone operation consists of removing the femoral head and leaving the upper end of the femur in the acetabular socket. This is a surprisingly successful operation and leaves the patient with a minimum amount of pain, though the hip is stiff and there is shortening of the leg. It can be considered as an option in patients who are not fit enough to undergo a full total hip replacement operation. Local anaesthetic hip block can be used to control pain in patients with severe OA but would not be appropriate in this patient as there are surgical options that would be expected to give a good result. There would be no point in attempting to replace the dynamic hip screw.

It has already been mentioned that trauma is an important risk factor and that the risk does not rise in old age. It is also important to distinguish juvenile nontraumatic avascular necrosis seen in children and young adults. Other important risk factors include:
- Corticosteroid treatment.
- Generalized severe arthrosclerosis.
- Any cause of peripheral vasospasm including Raynaud's disease.
- Decompression sickness (not to be ruled out in elderly active patients!).
- Sickle cell disease (usually presents in youth) and any cause of fat or air embolism.
- Mixed hyperlipidaemia.
- Excess alcohol consumption.
- Conditions of the hip joint capsule that can compromise blood supply such as infection, other forms of inflammation, and trauma.
- Metastatic disease to the hip joint.
- Pancreatic disease releasing lipolytic enzymes into the blood.
- Other haemoglobinopathies in addition to sickle cell disease.
- Patients receiving long-term haemodialysis.
- Any hypercoagulable state.

This is not an exhaustive list and it will be noted that some of these conditions are highly prevalent in elderly patients.

Patient 33

A 79-year-old man presented as an emergency with severe shortness of breath, intermittent confusion and inability to stand. He had a history of probable idiopathic pulmonary fibrosis and had suffered gradually increasing breathlessness over a 3-year period, though his shortness of breath had become progressively much worse over the last 3 days. He had a dry cough, recently worse, but produced little sputum. He had a 30 pack-year smoking history but gave up cigarettes about 8 years ago. His previous medical history consisted of hypertension, paroxysmal atrial fibrillation, and uncomplicated diverticular disease. Prior to presentation his drug regimen consisted of amiodarone 200 mg daily, amlodipine 10 mg daily, warfarin as per laboratory instruction, and Movicol 1 sachet daily. On examination he was afebrile and disorientated in time and place. His pulse was 100 bpm and irregularly irregular and heart auscultation revealed a quiet pansystolic murmur heard maximally at the cardiac apex and radiating to the left axilla. His BP was 110/70 mmHg lying down, respiratory rate 34 per minute, and there were mixed fine and coarse crackles audible throughout both lung fields but more so at the lung bases posteriorly. Examination of the abdomen, CNS, and skeleto-muscular system found no important abnormalities. On high flow oxygen supplementation his oxygen saturation was 91%.

Pulmonary function tests performed 1 year earlier had shown a restrictive lung defect with an FEV1 of 1.1 L (40% predicted). An ECG showed atrial fibrillation but no evidence of an acute myocardial infarction. Chest radiograph as in Figure 33.

Investigations (normal range)

Haemoglobin 10.9 g/dL (13–18)
MCV 79 f/L (80–96)
Total white cell count 10.8×10^9/L (4–11)
Neutrophil count 6.5×10^9/L (1.5–7)
Serum urea 9.1 mmol/L (2.5–7.5)
Serum creatinine 96 µmol/L (60–110)
Serum sodium 137 mmol/L (137–144)
Serum potassium 4.4 mmol/L (3.5–4.9)
INR 2.9

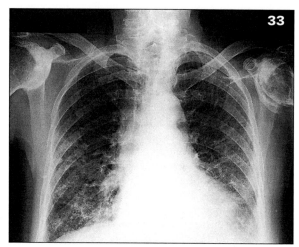

33 Plain chest radiograph taken on admission.

1 The most likely reason for this patient's recent deterioration is:
   A Pneumonia.
   B Heart failure.
   C Pulmonary embolism.
   D End-stage pulmonary fibrosis.
   E Exacerbation of COPD.

2 In addition to oxygen the best next acute treatment is:
   A Intravenous frusemide.
   B Intravenous digoxin.
   C Intravenous amoxicillin.
   D Intravenous dopamine.
   E Intravenous nitrate.

3 Comment on the patient's preadmission drug regimen. Would you consider any changes?

4 What is the most likely cause of his anaemia and how should it be investigated and managed?

Patient 33 Answers

---

1 B Heart failure.

The chest radiograph shows background chronic fibrotic change consistent with the diagnosis of pulmonary fibrosis. There is also some enlargement of the heart and softer interstitial shadowing, suggesting superimposed pulmonary oedema. Therefore, the most likely course of events in this patient is that the background pulmonary fibrosis has been complicated by an episode of acute heart failure. This is supported by the time course of the recent deterioration, the presence of relatively fast atrial fibrillation, the evidence of mitral incompetence, and the relatively low BP. The patient would also be predisposed to heart failure by his history of cigarette smoking and hypertension. Pneumonia cannot be absolutely ruled out but is unlikely as there is no leukocytosis or fever and the patient was not producing sputum. Pulmonary embolism is a possibility, although one would expect the onset to be more abrupt and it would be unlikely to occur in a patient who is taking warfarin. Furthermore, the radiographic changes are more supportive of superimposed heart failure than of pulmonary embolism. If the patient had proceeded to the end stages of pulmonary fibrosis, the history would be of more gradual worsening of the breathlessness. There is no strong evidence to suggest that the patient had COPD despite the smoking history, and the physical signs were not really those of COPD. In patients such as this where there is some doubt about the diagnosis, an urgent echocardiogram can be helpful.

---

2 A Intravenous frusemide.

The patient's deterioration and breathlessness is probably due to pulmonary oedema and this is likely to respond best to intravenous frusemide in the first instance as the patient is not critically hypotensive and has well-preserved renal function. A case could be made for adding intravenous digoxin to gain better control of the ventricular rate in this patient with atrial fibrillation. There is no indication for giving an antibiotic or an inotropic agent such as dopamine at this stage. Intravenous nitrate could be an important part of the overall treatment strategy for heart failure, though it would not be given before frusemide in these circumstances.

3 The patient was taking amiodarone prior to admission. This can cause pulmonary fibrosis so it will be important to ascertain whether the use of the drug had preceded the onset of the pulmonary fibrosis. If that was the case, it should be stopped and the atrial fibrillation controlled with an alternative drug such as digoxin (for rate control) or a beta-blocker to promote and sustain sinus rhythm. The patient is currently hypotensive so the amlodipine should be stopped and its long-term use reviewed at a later date. There is no indication to stop the warfarin for the time being.

4 The patient has a low haemoglobin and low MCV, suggesting iron deficiency. The most likely reason for this in the clinical context described is GI bleeding related to long-term warfarin treatment. Formal tests of the patient's iron status should be carried out and a decision needs to be made as to whether he should be investigated for specific sources of iron loss. In view of his severe cardiopulmonary condition, it is unlikely that he would be fit enough to undergo any surgical treatments. However, if his heart failure responds sufficiently well to treatment, a case could be made for performing upper and lower GI endoscopies to look for lesions that might be treated endoscopically (e.g. polyps or angiodysplasia) or with drugs (e.g. a peptic ulcer). An alternative, if the patient is thought to be too unwell for endoscopy, would be to give iron replacement therapy and a proton pump inhibitor to cover the possibility of upper GI bleeding.

Patient 34

An 81-year-old man was brought to hospital by his son because he had become acutely confused and was observed to have had several attacks of uncontrollable shivering. He had been complaining of pain in his perineum and the tip of his penis for about 2 days, and had noticed blood in his urine. For several months he had complained of a poor urinary stream but had not consulted his GP. He was otherwise in excellent health and was taking no medication. On examination, he had a body temperature of 38.4°C and was disorientated in time and place. His pulse was 96 bpm and regular, heart sounds normal, JVP normal, BP 150/90 mmHg, respiratory rate 16 per minute, with clear lung bases on auscultation. Examination of the abdomen revealed an enlarged bladder that was slightly tender and extended to 10 cm above the pubic symphasis. He was slightly tender on palpation of his renal angles. Rectal examination revealed a large, firm prostate. There were no significant abnormalities on examination of the CNS or skeleto-muscular system.

A chest radiograph was reported as normal, as was an ECG. Urine dipstick analysis could not be performed as the patient was not able to pass urine.

Investigations (normal range)

Haemoglobin 13.6 g/L (13–18)
MCV 88 fL (80–96)
Total white cell count 21.2×10^9/L (4–11)
Neutrophil count 19.8×10^9/L (1.5–7)
ESR 60 mm/h (<20)
Serum urea 31.0 mmol/L (2.5–7.5)
Serum creatinine 350 µmol/L (60–110)
Serum sodium 140 mmol/L (137–144)
Serum potassium 4.8 mmol/L (3.5–4.9)
Serum albumin 43 g/L (37–49)
Serum ALT 55 U/L (1–31)
Serum alkaline phosphatase 88 U/L (45–105)
Serum total bilirubin 12 µmol/L (1–22)
Serum corrected calcium 2.3 mmol/L (2.2–2.6)

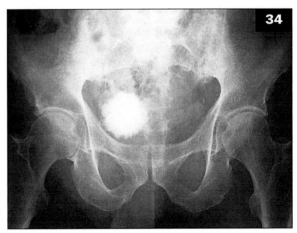

34 Plain radiograph of the abdomen taken during the patient's admission.

1 The most likely reason for this man's acute illness is:
  A Carcinoma of the prostate.
  B Urinary tract sepsis.
  C Multiple myeloma.
  D Transitional cell carcinoma of the bladder.
  E Prostatitis.

2 The most useful initial diagnostic test in this case is:
  A Measure PSA.
  B Plasma protein electrophoresis.
  C Catheter sample of urine for microbiology.
  D Abdominal ultrasound scan.
  E Urgent cystoscopy.

3 During this patient's admission a plain abdominal radiograph was performed (34). What is the abnormality on this radiograph? How might it be related to the patient's acute illness?

Patient 35

A 90-year-old man was admitted in a collapsed semi-conscious state. A medical student asks for instruction on the technique of hypodermoclysis as part of the patient's management.

1 What procedure does he want to learn?
  A Set up an intravenous infusion.
  B Set up a subcutaneous infusion.
  C Injecting a local anaesthetic.
  D Subcutaneous injection.
  E Suturing.

Patient 34 Answers

| 1 B Urinary tract sepsis. |

| 2 C Catheter sample of urine for microbiology. |

The most likely immediate reason for this man's acute presentation is urinary tract sepsis. A number of features support that as the most likely item on the differential diagnosis; the presentation with fever and rigors, the high neutrophil leukocytosis, the preceding obstructive lower urinary tract symptoms, and the slight tenderness suprapubically and in the renal angles. Carcinoma of the prostate remains a possibility as an underlying predisposing diagnosis in this man. There are no features to suggest underlying multiple myeloma; the moderately high ESR is most likely to be due to an acute-phase response in this context. Transitional cell carcinoma of the bladder usually presents with haematuria, though, like carcinoma of the prostate, it can be a predisposing factor in urinary tract sepsis. Acute prostatitis is a possibility in this patient and, indeed, prostatic infection may be part of a more generalized urinary tract septic state. However, most patients with prostatitis present subacutely with dysuria and pain at the base of the penis at the end of micturition.

In the early stage of this illness it is important to try to establish a microbiological diagnosis. The patient is unable to pass urine and has evidence of compromised renal function, so a catheter will need to be inserted as part of the management for that aspect of this patient's condition. At the same time a catheter specimen of urine can be obtained for microbiological analysis including culture and sensitivity. Measuring PSA as a screening test for carcinoma of prostate is unreliable in the presence of acute lower urinary tract sepsis, which can cause the PSA to be high. Plasma protein electrophoresis is not indicated in this case. An abdominal ultrasound scan is justified because of the possibility of an obstructive uropathy in this patient (obstructive symptoms, presentation with acute retention, and compromised renal function) but would not necessarily be the first investigation to be done. Cystoscopy would not normally be performed until the obstructed state had been relieved and sepsis controlled.

3 The abnormality on the plain abdominal radiograph is a large bladder stone. Such stones predispose a patient to lower urinary tract infection and can cause dysuric symptoms or even obstruction. They can also be totally asymptomatic. Large bladder stones are now relative uncommon in the UK. Patients found to have a bladder stone should be referred to an urologist for further management.

Patient 35 Answer

| 1 B Set up a subcutaneous infusion. |

Hypodermoclysis is the subcutaneous infusion of fluids. It is a useful and easy hydration technique suitable for mildly to moderately dehydrated adult patients, especially elderly subjects who are restless or have fragile veins. The method is considered safe and does not cause any serious complications. The most frequent adverse effect is mild subcutaneous oedema that can be treated by local massage or a change in the infusion site. Infection is usually localized to the site of the needle. The indications and contraindications of hypodermoclysis are given in *Table 35*.

Table 35 *Indications and contraindications for hypodermoclysis*

Indications
Treatment and prevention of mild to moderate dehydration in patients with:
- Poor oral intake
- Diarrhoea, diuretics
- Poor venous access with difficulty administering enteral or parenteral nutrition
- Drowsiness, confusion
- Dysphagia

Terminal phase of life:
- To infuse opioid analgesics and other drugs (with fluids if appropriate)
- At the request of the patient
- To help reduce symptoms of dry mouth, constipation, confusion

To infuse an amino acid solution to limit malnutrition
Contraindications
- Shock, circulatory failure, or severe dehydration
- Fluid overload states
- Bleeding disorders

Patient 36

An 88-year-old woman was referred to the Outpatient Department by her GP. She had complained of increasing tiredness, shortness of breath on exertion, headache, and low back pain. The GP found her to be anaemic with a haemoglobin of 8.9 g/dL and plasma viscosity of 1.91 mPa/s (1.5–1.72). In clinic she described progressive symptoms over a number of weeks, though she had felt entirely well 3 months earlier. Her only significant previous medical history was of a hysterectomy performed at the age of 42 and a left elective total hip replacement at the age of 80 for OA. She was taking no medication other than occasional paracetamol and lived independently. On examination she was pale and dyspnoeic after walking into the clinic. There was no lymphadenopathy. Pulse was 90 bpm regular, heart sounds normal, BP 145/90 mmHg with no signs of cardiac failure. Respiratory rate settled to 16 per minute after 5 minutes rest and there were no abnormalities on auscultation of the chest, though the patient did have some tenderness on the left side of the thorax, postero-laterally. Abdominal examination was normal. Skeleto-muscular examination revealed tenderness of the spine on direct pressure at the level of L1 and minor osteoarthrotic changes in the knees. The patient indicated an area close to her occiput which appeared to be the centre of her headache and it was found that her skull was painful on direct pressure in that position.

A chest radiograph was reported as normal. Her skull radiograph is shown (**36**). There were no abnormalities on her ECG and a routine specimen of urine showed moderate protein but no other abnormalities.

> *Investigations (normal range)*
>
> Haemoglobin 8.4 g/dL (11.5–16.5)
> MCV 94 fL (80–96)
> Total white cell count 4.1 × 10⁹/L (4–11)
> Platelet count 120 × 10⁹/L (150–400)
> ESR 94 mm/h (<30)
> Serum sodium 139 mmol/L (137–144)
> Serum potassium 5.5 mmol/L (3.5–4.9)
> Serum urea 29.4 mmol/L (2.5–7.5)
> Serum creatinine 335 µmol/L (60–110)
> Serum total protein 84g/L (61–76)
> Serum albumin 33g/L (37–49)
> Serum total bilirubin 9 µmol/L (1–22)
> Serum corrected calcium 3.2 mmol/L (2.2–2.6)
> Serum alkaline phosphatase 250 U/L (45–105)
> Plasma parathyroid hormone
>   1.1 pmol/L(0.9–5.4)

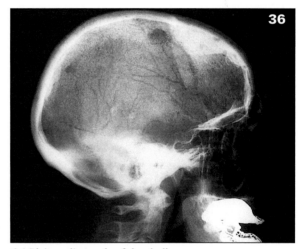

36 Plain radiograph of the skull.

1 The most likely diagnosis in this patient is:
  A Waldenstrom's macroglobulinaemia.
  B Plasmacytoma.
  C Multiple myeloma.
  D MGUS.
  E Disseminated lymphoma.

2 Further investigations showed the presence of a paraprotein band on plasma protein electrophoresis. Based on that, and the other information available, which of the following investigations would best confirm the most likely diagnosis?
  A Bone marrow aspiration.
  B Imaging-guided biopsy of a skull lesion.
  C Assessment of glomerular filtration rate.
  D Quantification of urinary Bence-Jones protein.
  E CT head scan.

3 From the information available, broadly assess the patient's prognosis.

Patient 36 Answers

1 C Multiple myeloma.

2 D Quantification of urinary Bence-Jones protein.

Multiple myeloma is the most likely. This is supported by the presence of several lytic lesions in the skull, the anaemia and renal impairment, and the high plasma viscosity and ESR. Waldenstrom's macroglobulanaemia is an important cause of a high ESR and hyperviscocity, though it is unusual for there to be significant suppression of bone marrow or renal impairment, to the extent seen in this patient. Furthermore, discrete lytic bone lesions would not be expected. A plasmacytoma can cause a lytic bone lesion but is usually solitary and though it might secrete a low amplitude paraprotein, there would not usually be any other systemic effect. By definition, this patient does not have a MGUS because of the presence of multiple system involvement. MGUS is diagnosed when a paraprotein is found on plasma protein electrophoresis, usually of relatively low amplitude, and there is no evidence of destructive involvement of other systems. Some lymphomas secrete monoclonal proteins but would not cause the other features seen in this patient.

The patient already has two of the criteria required to make the diagnosis of multiple myeloma: the presence of a paraprotein in the serum, and lytic lesions in bone. The demonstration of Bence-Jones proteins in urine, particularly if these are plentiful, secures the diagnosis. Bone marrow aspiration in patients with multiple myeloma often demonstrates the presence of excessive plasma cells, though this is not invariable. There is no indication for attempting to biopsy one of the lytic lesions. This would show infiltration of bone with plasma cells but does not advance the position diagnostically. This patient's glomerular filtration rate will certainly be reduced and it may be necessary to measure it to track the renal impairment. However, it is not a diagnostic test in multiple myeloma. A CT head scan would provide no further specific information regarding the myeloma lesions in the skull.

3 The patient described has a number of adverse prognostic features including hypercalcaemia, a raised alkaline phosphatase (suggesting hepatic involvement as bone destruction by myeloma does not usually cause a rise in the serum alkaline phosphatase), and a low serum albumin. The suppression of haemopoeisis and renal involvement are also adverse prognostic findings. Although the information was not given in this patient, the presence of a very high amplitude monoclonal protein band on electrophoresis, within the context described in this patient, would also be broadly associated with a worse prognosis.

Tutorial

Multiple myeloma is a relatively common condition in old age with an incidence that rises with age steeply after the age of 70. MGUS is also common in this age group. By definition, elderly patients with MGUS do not require specific treatment, though their condition should be monitored. Elderly patients with multiple myeloma may not need to be treated with chemotherapy if they are asymptomatic and do not have rapidly progressive impairment of haemopoeisis and/or renal function. Some older patients do benefit from chemotherapy, though the general consensus among haematologists is that they tend to do better with relatively low-dose monochemotherapy, rather than multiple drug regimens. Very frail elderly patients with advanced multiple myeloma do not appear to benefit from chemotherapy and should be offered good quality palliative management. In most cases these therapeutic decisions should be made in conjunction with haematologists, to decide the best option for any individual.

Patient 37

A 77-year-old woman was referred for urgent domiciliary assessment. Her GP was concerned about a painful ulcer that had appeared on the patient's right leg over a period of several days. The patient had a long history of RA and had been using an electric wheelchair for about 4 years. She was able to transfer herself from the wheelchair into her bed, or to the toilet, alone but with difficulty. Her other previous medical history included childhood rheumatic heart disease for which she had received a mitral valve replacement 6 years ago. A fall had resulted in a fracture of the neck of the right femur that was treated operatively with an Austin Moore hemiarthroplasty. Her medication consisted of paracetamol 1 g three times daily, methotrexate 10 mg once weekly, folic acid 5 mg daily, warfarin variable dose depending on INR, and digoxin 125 μg daily. On examination her temperature was 36.8°C, she was slightly pale but there was no lymphadenopathy. She was fully alert with an AMTS of 10/10 and normal bedside screening tests for frontal executive function. Her pulse was 78 bpm irregularly irregular, auscultation of her heart revealed a prosthetic 1st heart sound and normal 2nd heart sound, BP 135/85 mmHg, respiratory rate 16 per minute, and a few coarse crackles could be heard at both lung bases which cleared on coughing. Abdominal examination was normal and, in particular, there was no splenomegaly. Examination of the skin revealed appropriate age-related changes and no rash. Skeleto-muscular system examination showed extensive rheumatoid arthritic changes in the hands but no evidence to suggest an acute flare-up of that condition. There was a small effusion in the left knee and in both shoulder joints, though those joints were not tender. Her feet were warm and all peripheral pulses were palpable. She had no sign of varicose veins and there was very little ankle oedema. An ulcer was present on the right leg (**37a**).

A radiograph of the patient's hands is shown in Figure **37b**.

Investigations (normal range)

Haemoglobin 10.5 g/dL (11.5–16.5)
MCV 81 fL (80–96)
Total white cell count 4.4×10^9/L (4–11)
Neutrophil count 3.8×10^9/L (1.5–4)
ESR 64 mm/h (<30)
Serum urea, creatinine, sodium, potassium
    all within normal range
Serum albumin 36 g/L (37–49)
Serum total bilirubin 19 μmol/L (1–22)
Serum ALT 42 U/L (5–35)
Serum AST 39 U/L (1–31)
Fasting plasma glucose 5.5 mmol/L (3–6)
Plasma thyroxine 84 nmol/L (58–174)
Serum CRP 44 mg/L (<10)
Plasma protein electrophoresis diffuse
    increase in IgG, IgM
Rheumatoid factor 84 kU/L (<30)
Antinuclear factor positive
Antidouble-stranded DNA antibody 150 U/mL
    (<73)
ANCA negative
INR 3.9 (target range 3.5–4.5)

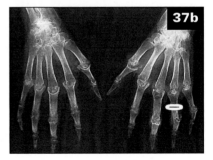

37a Painful ulcer on the right leg.

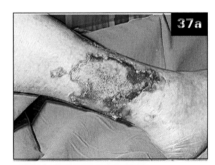

37b Plain radiograph of the patient's hands.

1 The most likely cause of this patient's ulcer is:
  A Venous insufficiency.   D Pyoderma
  B Pyogenic cellulitis.   gangrenosum.
  C Arterial insufficiency.   E Systemic vasculitis.

2 The most prudent next step in the immediate management of this patient is:
  A Intravenous broad-spectrum antibiotic treatment.
  B Topical antibacterial dressings.
  C Oral colchicine.
  D Oral azothiaprine.
  E Oral corticosteroids.

3 What are the most important aspects of supportive care for this patient?

4 Describe the radiological features seen in Figure **37b**.

Patient 37 Answers

> **1 D** Pyoderma gangrenosum.

The most likely lesion in this case is pyoderma gangrenosum. This is supported by the rapid onset of the ulcer, its slightly scalloped edges, deep basal slough, and inflamed-looking rim. The patient also has a risk factor for pyoderma gangrenosum in that she has sero-positive rheumatoid disease. The appearance is not really that of a venous insufficiency ulcer even though the position could suggest that condition. There is no history of venous insufficiency in this patient and the mode of onset and appearance does not support that diagnosis. A cellulitis leading to abscess formation and ulceration would usually be accompanied by an extensive area of cutaneous erythema, a high white cell count, and fever. The patient had warm feet and intact foot pulses so arterial insufficiency is most unlikely. A thromboembolic event in the foot would not normally cause ulceration in this position and would in any case usually present with a blackened part and dry gangrene. Vasculitis cannot be ruled out, though focal vasculitis causing a large ulcer, such as this, is very unusual. In a patient with a more generalized vasculitis, there would usually be other physical signs and in most cases there would be some degree of renal impairment.

> **2 E** Oral corticosteroids.

Predicated on the answer to Question 1, the most appropriate immediate treatment in this patient would be high-dose corticosteroids, probably starting at at least 60 mg of prednisolone daily. There is no indication for antibiotics since there is no good supporting evidence of sepsis. Similarly, there is nothing to be gained by applying a topical antibacterial dressing. Colchicine is effective to some extent in pyoderma gangrenosum. Although the aetiology of the condition is not fully understood, it is now classified with other auto-inflammatory conditions such as familial Mediterranean fever and responds to colchicine through the effect of that drug on neutrophil chemotaxis. Azothiaprine is also sometimes used as an adjunctive treatment for pyoderma gangrenosum, though the evidence of efficacy is not firmly established. Most patients with pyoderma gangrenosum will respond rapidly to corticosteroid treatment. In many patients that response is sufficiently dramatic to be considered as further confirmation of the diagnosis.

3 The patient described in this case has maintained her independence by using an electric wheelchair and preserving her ability to transfer from the wheelchair to her bed and toilet. Therefore, when managing this patient, it is vital to try to preserve that degree of mobility by starting supporting physical therapies as soon as possible. A prolonged and unnecessary period of bed rest would almost certainly rob the patient of her remaining independence. The ulcer requires careful dressings to avoid secondary infection and there must be adequate analgesia. The potential side-effects of steroid therapy need to be addressed, including glucose intolerance, salt and water retention, and a further reduction in proximal muscle power. If there is to be prolonged treatment with corticosteroids, the patient should receive prophylaxis to reduce the progression of osteoporosis, including calcium and vitamin D, and a bisphosphonate. This will be particularly important for a patient who is still walking independently. Once the ulcer has responded to treatment, an attempt should be made to reduce the corticosteroid dose as quickly as possible. In some patients who require longer-term maintenance corticosteroid treatment, the side-effects can be reduced by giving intermittent intravenous methylprednisolone.

4 The radiographs of the hands in this patient show typical moderately severe rheumatoid changes including bony erosions in the joints, lucencies in the bone adjacent to joints, and deformities.

> ### Tutorial
>
> As the pathogenic processes causing pyoderma gangrenosum have become clearer, a number of potential new treatments has emerged. As well as systemic corticosteroids there has been some success with high-potency topical corticosteroids and a number of drugs that modify immune sequences such as tacrolimus, chromalin sodium, and 5-aminosalicylic acid. As the role of TNF in autoinflammatory conditions has been established, there has been successful treatments given with TNF-alpha inhibitors, such as infliximab, and a wide range of more well-established drugs that suppress inflammation such as dapsone, thalidomide, and biological agents that modify cytokine responses. *Table 37* presents diseases associated with pyoderma gangrenosum.

Table 37 *Diseases associated with pyoderma gangrenosum*

- Sero-positive and sero-negative rheumatoid disease
- Inflammatory bowel disease
- Leukaemia and proleukaemia states (particularly myeloid leukaemias)
- Monoclonal gammopathies (particularly multiple myeloma)

- Less common associations:
  - Polyarthritis
  - Chronic hepatitides
- Other immunological conditions (SLE)
- In some patients there is no identifiable predisposing condition

Patient 38

An 82-year-old woman was referred urgently by her GP. For 2 days she had become unable to walk, complaining of painful feet. She had a 12-year history of hypertension, atrial fibrillation for 8 years, and stable intermittent claudication (at 100 m) for 2 years. She had a 40 pack-year smoking history and still smoked about 10 cigarettes/day. Her medication was digoxin 125 µg daily, bendroflumethiazide 2.5 mg daily, and aspirin 150 mg daily. On examination she was afebrile, in obvious pain but not confused (AMTS 9/10). Her pulse was 60 bpm and irregularly irregular, JVP normal, heart sounds normal, BP 160/95 mmHg. Her respiratory rate was 14 per minute and there were quiet expiratory rhonchi audible at the lung bases as she breathed down to residual volume. Abdominal examination revealed an expansile mass in the umbilical region. Her femoral, popliteal, posterior tibial, and dorsalis pedis pulses were all palpable in both legs. Arterial brachio-pedal indices were 0.91 on the left and 0.94 on the right. Both feet had the appearance shown in Figure **38a**.

A chest radiograph showed slight hyperinflation but was otherwise normal. An echocardiogram revealed good left ventricular function, a left atrial diameter of 4.0 cm (normal <3.5) and no evidence of thrombus in any cardiac chamber. An abdominal ultrasound scan showed a 6.5 cm diameter infrarenal abdominal aortic aneurysm. A routine specimen of urine showed slight proteinuria but was otherwise normal.

Investigations (normal range)

Haemoglobin 12.4 g/dL (11.5–16.5)
Total white cell count 10.9 × 10^9/L (4–11)
Neutrophil count 7.0 × 10^9/L (1.5–7)
Eosinophil count 1.1 × 10^9/L (0.04–0.4)
Platelet count 230 × 10^9/L (150–400)
ESR 64 mm/h (<30)
Serum urea 10.1 mmol/L (2.5–7.5)
Serum creatinine 90 µmol/L (60–110)
Serum albumin 44g/L (37–49)
Serum ALT 19 U/L (5–35)
Serum alkaline phosphatase 81 U/L (45–105)
Plasma glucose 5.2 mmol/L (3–6)
D-dimer concentration 0.7 mg/L (<0.5)

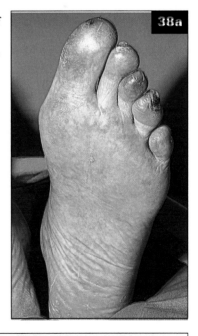

38a Photograph of the patient's left foot. Both feet had this appearance.

1 Which of the following diagnoses best explains the clinical presentation:
  A Thromboembolism from the left atrium.
  B Thromboembolism from the aorta.
  C Femoral artery stenosis.
  D Cholesterol crystal embolism.
  E Arteriosclerotic small vessel disease.

2 How can the diagnosis be confirmed?

3 Summarize the treatment and prognosis for this patient.

Patient 38 Answers

---

1 D Cholesterol crystal embolism.

The most likely diagnosis is cholesterol crystal embolism. This is supported by the sudden onset of bilateral peripheral small vessel obstruction in the presence of palpable pulses. The patient is predisposed to cholesterol crystal embolization by the presence of macrovascular disease (in this case an aortic aneurysm) and a number of vascular risk factors including hypertension and smoking. The presence of an eosinophilia is also typical of cholesterol crystal embolism, though that finding is not invariable. A small rise in D-dimer is consistent with the diagnosis.

Thromboembolism from the left atrium would be expected, in most cases, to cause a unilateral arterial obstruction and it is more likely that a larger vessel would be obstructed by a thrombus arising from a heart chamber. This also applies to thromboembolism arising from the surface of the aorta. Femoral artery stenosis would not normally present acutely and in any case would tend to be asymmetrical and be associated with diminished or absent pulses in the lower limb. Arteriosclerotic small vessel disease would be expected in a hypertensive smoker with macrovascular disease but is an insidious and gradual condition, therefore unlikely to present in this dramatic fashion. The appearance of the feet in Figure **38a** is also highly typical of cholesterol crystal embolization.

2 The only certain way to make the diagnosis is to obtain a histological specimen and demonstrate the presence of cholesterol crystals in small arterioles. This can sometimes be seen on renal biopsy in patients with renal involvement or in amputation specimens of the foot or toes, or at postmortem. A characteristic appearance is seen (**38b**), whereby splinter-shaped clefts are left in the histological specimen after fixing the material and dissolving out the cholesterol crystals.

3 Cholesterol crystal embolism carries a poor prognosis. In patients diagnosed antemortem, the mortality in some series has been as high as 50%. If the cholesterol crystals are released from a ruptured atherosclerotic plaque above the level of the renal arteries, there is almost invariably an abrupt onset of acute renal failure, which carries a high mortality rate in this group of patients, many of whom have other vascular co-morbidities. Patients with infra-renal crystal release have a somewhat better prognosis, though it is not uncommon for toes or feet to be lost. The long-term prognosis is also poor as the patients remain prone to further release of cholesterol crystals from plaques in the aorta.

Treatment is difficult. There are no satisfactory specific treatments available. Supportive therapies including dialysis, control of sepsis, and optimization of BP are important. The place of anticoagulation is uncertain despite the fact that some patients develop disseminated intravascular coagulation. Most studies have shown no benefit and some have shown an adverse effect of anticoagulation in this context. Generally speaking, invasive investigations and surgical procedures that might further disrupt cholesterol plaques should be avoided.

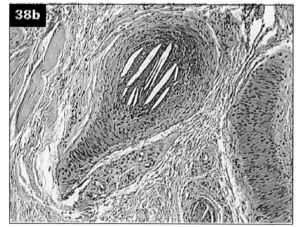

38b Photomicrograph showing characteristic 'clefts' of cholesterol crystal embolism.

Tutorial

Any downstream organ can be damaged by the release of cholesterol crystals, depending on the site of release. There is case report evidence in the literature of patients dying from cholesterol crystal embolization to the pancreas, GI tract, and brain, as well as the more usual sites of kidneys and lower limbs. The most important risk factors are an age of greater than 60, male sex, hypertension, hypercholesterolaemia, smoking, and diabetes mellitus. Recent cardiac catheterization or other invasive arterial procedures constitute an acute risk factor. The majority of patients presenting with cholesterol crystal embolism already have an established diagnosis of cerebrovascular, cardiovascular, or peripheral vascular disease, or a mixture thereof.

Patient 39

A 90-year-old woman was brought to hospital by her daughter. The patient had felt slightly unwell for about 4 days, was reluctant to eat and was intermittently confused. On the day of admission she had complained of sore legs and feet and her daughter noticed several large blisters on both legs below the knees. She mentioned that a similar blister had appeared a few weeks earlier but it had burst within hours and settled; it had been thought at that time to be due to a burn from a hot water bottle. Her previous medical history included mild Parkinson's disease, a right Austin Moore hemi-arthroplasty for a fractured neck of femur, and the removal of several dysplastic colonic polyps at colonoscopy after investigation for iron deficiency anaemia. Her medication consisted of ferrous sulphate 400 mg twice daily, paracetamol 1 g as required, calcium and vitamin D one tablet daily, and weekly alendronate. On examination she had a temperature of 37.8°C and her AMTS was 6/10. GCS was 15/15. Her pulse was 86 bpm and regular, BP 140/80 mmHg with normal heart sounds and no signs of cardiac failure. Her respiratory rate was 16 per minute and examination of the chest was normal. There were no abnormalities on examination of the abdomen, other than one small collapsed blister close to the umbilicus. Examination of the rest of her skin revealed several large, thin-walled, slack blisters on both legs, some of which had already collapsed and drained a clear fluid. Two more blisters were found on the left arm and one small one close to the left shoulder posteriorly. Within about 12 hours the blisters on her legs had been through a phase of coalescence and had all ruptured and drained. It was noticed that the skin close to the edge of some of the blisters had a normal appearance but that the epidermis could be slid across the underlying dermis. A photograph taken the day after her admission can be seen in Figure 39.

Her renal, liver and thyroid function tests were all normal and a routine specimen of urine was negative for blood and protein. A chest radiograph was reported as normal.

Investigations (normal range)

Haemoglobin 12.1 g/L (11.5–16.5)
Total white cell count 10.1×10^9/L (4–11)
Neutrophil count 8.5×10^9/L (1.5–7)
ESR 55 mm/h (<30)

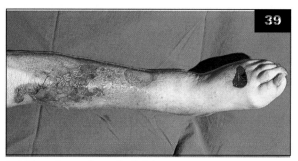

39 Blistering rash on the left leg.

1 Which of the following is the most likely diagnosis:
   A Toxic epidermolysis.
   B Erythema multiforme.
   C Pemphigus vulgaris.
   D Bullous pemphigoid.
   E Blistering drug eruption.

2 How can the diagnosis be confirmed?

3 In this patient, the most important next line of treatment is:
   A Corticosteroids.
   B Antibiotics.
   C Intravenous fluids.
   D Plasmaphoresis.
   E Anti-TNF-alpha.

4 Comment on any unusual aspects of the presentation in this patient.

Patient 39 Answers

1 C Pemphigus vulgaris.	3 A Corticosteroids.

The most likely diagnosis is pemphigus vulgaris. This is supported by the presence of large painful thin-walled blisters arising from otherwise normal-looking skin. The presence of loose epidermis beyond the edge of the bullae (Nikolsky's sign) strongly supports the diagnosis. A patient with toxic epidermolysis due to, for example, staphylococcal infection, would be expected to be more ill than this patient, with a higher fever and leukocytosis. There is also usually more erythema associated with the formation of blisters due to infection. Nevertheless, it should be borne in mind as an important differential diagnosis in a patient presenting this way. The lesions do not look like those of typical erythema multiforme and in this patient there were no mucosal features (though mucosal involvement is sometimes seen in patients with pemphigus vulgaris). A fixed drug eruption is always a possibility in a patient with this type of presentation, though the drugs being taken by the patient in this case are very rarely associated with blistering skin eruptions. Bullous pemphigoid is an important part of the differential diagnosis. However, in that condition the blisters have a thicker wall and are much less likely to burst spontaneously. Furthermore, Nikolsky's sign would be negative.

2 The diagnosis can be confirmed by demonstrating the presence of pemphigus autoantibodies (antidesmogline antibodies) and/or demonstrating fluorescent antihuman IgG antibody uptake in the subepidermal layer of a biopsy specimen taken from the edge of the blister. In bullous pemphigoid, immunofluorescent staining demonstrates uptake in the basement membrane zone and antibody attachment at the level of the lamina lucida. Distinct bullous pemphigoid antibodies can also be demonstrated on serological testing.

The patient was quite unwell and needed treatment to suppress the formation of further blisters. This is best achieved by giving corticosteroids at a fairly high dose (60–100 mg/day prednisolone). This will arrest the disease and allow the skin to heal in the majority of patients. There was no indication for antibiotics in this patient since there was no clear evidence of infection. The patient had no signs of being in a dehydrated or hypovolaemic state so fluids could be given orally. Theoretically, plasmaphoresis should help to suppress blister formation by removing circulating pemphigus autoantibody, though it is rarely used in this condition because of the good response to corticosteroids and the evidence for its efficacy is weak. There is no evidence to support the first-line use of anti-TNF-alpha for pemphigus. The long-term management of the majority of patients with pemphigus is best done in conjunction with a dermatologist so as to get the best disease control with a minimum exposure to corticosteroids and other anti-inflammatory medications. In patients where there is any uncertainty about the diagnosis, specialist help should be sought.

4 The unusual features in this patient include the age of onset (patients with pemphigus vulgaris usually present in middle age rather than old age, whereas those with bullous pemphigoid more commonly present in old age), and the distribution of the lesions (the more peripheral distribution is more typical of bullous pemphigoid). However, the diagnosis of pemphigus vulgaris was confirmed in this patient serologically.

Tutorial

Some patients with infrequent, minimal and trivial bullous pemphigoid, and occasionally pemphigus vulgaris, can be managed without long-term immunosuppressive treatment. The logic to this is that the side-effects of treatment in such patients can be more detrimental than the disease. This is rarely likely to be the case in pemphigus vulgaris but is commonly the right course of action in bullous pemphigoid when the patient is suffering occasional limited blistering once or twice a year. In some patients, bullous pemphigoid or pemphigus vulgaris can be the presenting features of an underlying neoplasm so it is prudent to investigate further if there are any other features to suggest an underlying malignant process.

Patient 40

A 78-year-old woman wandered into her neighbour's house in a bewildered state. She lived alone and independently and had been observed to be entirely well the previous day. She took no medication and her previous medical history was not known. The patient's neighbour called in the GP who found an axillary temperature of 36.9°C and made a provisional diagnosis of a minor stroke based on the confusional state and the presence of probable word-finding difficulty. Four hours later at the hospital a rigor was observed, at which time a rectal temperature was 39.4°C, the patient was increasingly confused, and had cold hands and feet. There was no lymphadenopathy or rash noted. Her pulse was 100 bpm and regular, heart sounds normal, BP 120/70 mmHg. Examination of the chest revealed a respiratory rate of 18 per minute with no abnormal findings on auscultation. The patient's abdomen was slightly tender in all quadrants and in the renal angles. There were no focal neurological signs and her GCS score was 13/15. A routine specimen of urine was slightly positive for blood and protein. A provisional diagnosis of UTI was made and the patient was treated with intravenous amoxicillin. Over the subsequent three hours the patient's GCS fell progressively from 13 to 10, at which time an urgent CT head scan showed no abnormalities. She remained febrile and a scanty nonblanching rash appeared (**40**).

A chest radiograph was normal and an ECG showed sinus tachycardia but no other abnormalities. Blood cultures were set up.

Investigations (normal range)

Haemoglobin 13.1 g/dL (11.5–16.5)
Total white cell count 18.1 × 10^9/L (4–11)
Neutrophil count 17.2 × 10^9/L (1.5–7)
Serum urea 14.2 mmol/L (2.5–7.5)
Serum creatinine 78 mmol/L (60–110)
Serum sodium 139 mmol/L (137–144)
Serum potassium 4.4 mmol/L (3.5–4.9)
Serum ALT 71 U/L (5–35)
Serum total bilirubin 8 mmol/L (1–22)
Serum alkaline phosphatase 50 U/L (45–105)
Oxygen saturation 95%

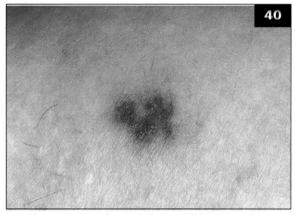

40 Close up view of a single lesion of the nonblanching rash.

1 The most likely diagnosis is:
  A Meningococcal septicaemia.
  B Pneumococcal septicaemia.
  C Gram-negative sepsis.
  D Systemic vasculitis.
  E *Salmonella* septicaemia.

2 The best management strategy, while awaiting further investigation results, is:
  A To continue with the amoxicillin.
  B Add gentamicin to the amoxicillin.
  C Change to ceftriaxone.
  D Change to intravenous vancomycin and trimethoprim.
  E Change to ciprofloxacin.

3 Comment on the finding of a temperature of 36.9°C prior to admission and on the provisional diagnosis of UTI made at the time of admission.

Patient 40 Answers

1 A Meningococcal septicaemia.

2 C Change to ceftriaxone.

The most likely diagnosis in this patient is meningococcal septicaemia. It is not possible to be absolutely certain, though the diagnosis at this stage is supported by the fact that the patient was in good health until the day before her presentation (meningococcal sepsis tends to come on abruptly and can occur in otherwise entirely well individuals), the high fever and leukocytosis, and the presence of a purpuric rash. The absence of meningitic signs in this patient does not rule out the possibility of associated meningococcal meningitis. Pneumococcal septicaemia can also be very abrupt in onset, though most patients will have some evidence of focal pneumococcal infection such as lobar pneumonia. Pneumococcal septicaemia is not normally associated with a purpuric rash. The same applies to Gram-negative sepsis; this may present with a rapidly advancing acute septic clinical picture, though in most patients a focus for Gram-negative infection can be identified, such as definite UTI, cholecystitis, or diverticulitis. Nevertheless, some patients with Gram-negative septicaemia will present with no obvious portal of entry. Systemic vasculitis can cause a purpuric rash but would normally be more subacute or even chronic in its presentation, and is unlikely to be associated with such a high fever and leukocytosis. *Salmonella* septicaemia, usually due to *S. enteritidis* in temperate climates, can be an overwhelmingly severe illness mimicking enteric fever. There is usually, but not invariably, an associated *Salmonella* GI infection. The associated rash is usually a scanty pink macular rash, which does blanch on pressure.

Because of the high likelihood of meningococcal disease, and the possibility of associated meningococcal meningitis in this patient, it would be sensible to choose ceftriaxone from the options presented. A lumbar puncture to confirm or rule out associated meningitis would be good practice and can be performed safely in this patient because the CT head scan has ruled out abnormalities of intracranial pressure. Continuing amoxicillin on its own would be inadequate in this context, particularly since the patient has continued to deteriorate after amoxicillin was started. Adding gentamicin would cover a large range of bacteria but would probably be suboptimal in this particular patient. Intravenous vancomycin and trimethoprim would normally be reserved for the management of highly resistant strains of *Staphylococcus aureus* so are not indicated here, and ciprofloxacin would not be the best choice for a probable meningococcal disease. It is not possible to be dogmatic about antibiotic options so clinicians should always follow their locally agreed antibiotic policies and, where necessary, take microbiological advice.

3 The initial axillary temperature of 36.9°C measured in the patient's home was almost certainly an underestimate. In older patients the axilla requires up to 10 minutes to reach a stable temperature after closure and so is rarely a practical means of assessing core body temperature. Older patients often have relatively modest pyrexial responses to infection so axillary temperature is particularly likely to miss a low-grade fever. There was no really good evidence to support the diagnosis of UTI. The patient did not have any obvious dysuric symptoms and the mild generalized tenderness in the abdomen is a frequent finding in patients with septicaemia. Furthermore, the urine on routine testing showed small amounts of blood and protein, which would not be unusual in an older patient, particularly if febrile, and is not strong supporting evidence of UTI. The temptation to explain away acute confusional states in elderly patients by making the unsupported diagnosis of UTI is widespread but must be resisted. In the patient described in this case, her only hope of survival lay in proper assessment, appropriate investigation, and the prompt use of antibiotics. The search for a correct diagnosis can be delayed by the inexcusable use of pseudo-diagnoses of convenience.

Patient 41

A 77-year-old man was referred by his GP. He had been treated for three culture-positive symptomatic UTIs in the preceding 2 months, each caused by coliform organisms and responding to antibiotics. There was also a history of a poor appetite and 6 kg of weight loss over the same time period. More recently, the patient had complained of persistent and worsening mid dorsal back pain, which was not relieved by paracetamol. He was taking no medications. He did not smoke, or drink alcohol. Examination revealed an afebrile patient with no lymphadenopathy or abnormal skin signs. His pulse was 100 bpm and regular, heart sounds normal, BP 155/85 mmHg, respiratory rate 20 per minute with no abnormal signs on auscultation of the chest. Examination of the abdomen and CNS was normal and on examination of the skeleto-muscular system the only abnormality was mild tenderness over the sacrum.

An ECG showed sinus tachycardia but was otherwise normal. A radiograph of his lumbar spine is shown in Figure 41. A routine specimen of urine was positive for blood but otherwise negative.

Investigations (normal range)

Haemoglobin 9.1 g/dL (13–18)
MCV 92 fL (80–96)
Total white cell count 8.2×10^9/L (4–11)
Neutrophil count 6.7×10^9/L (1.5–7)
Serum urea 15.9 mmol/L (2.5–7.5)
Serum creatinine 103 µmol/L (60–110)
Serum sodium 145 mmol/L (137–144)
Serum potassium 4.6 mmol/L (3.5–4.9)
Serum corrected calcium 3.4 mmol/L (2.2–2.6)
Serum phosphate 1.1 mmol/L (0.8–1.4)
Serum alkaline phosphatase 210 U/L (45–105)
Serum ALT 27 U/L (5–35)
Serum bilirubin 16 µmol/L (1–22)
Serum albumin 34 g/L (37–49)

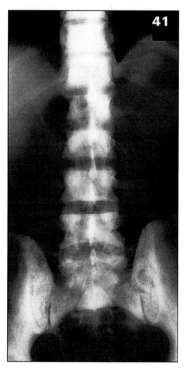

41 Plain radiograph of the lumbar and sacral spine.

1 The most useful next test for diagnostic purposes is:
   A Plasma protein electrophoresis.
   B Bone alkaline phosphatase isoenzyme.
   C PSA.
   D Serum parathyroid hormone.
   E Serum aluminium.

2 The most sensible first-line treatment for the hypercalcaemia is:
   A Intravenous pamidronate.
   B Subcutaneous calcitonin.
   C Intravenous frusemide.
   D Intravenous fluids.
   E Oral strontium ranelate.

3 What is the most likely reason for the anaemia?

4 What further tests might be needed?

Patient 41 Answers

---

1 C PSA.

The patient has presented with dysuric symptoms, has haematuria, and the radiograph of the spine shows extensive sclerosis. This all suggests underlying carcinoma of the prostate in an elderly man so the most useful immediate test would be to measure PSA. Plasma protein electrophoresis is not likely to be helpful in this case. It would probably show a polyclonal increase in Igs associated with the recent UTIs. Myeloma usually causes bone lysis rather than sclerosis. There is little point in identifying bone alkaline phosphatase isoenzyme in this patient as there is a reason to expect the alkaline phosphatase to be of bone origin. Furthermore, there are no other significant abnormalities of liver function. Parathyroid hormone assay would be a sensible investigation in patients with otherwise unexplained hypercalcaemia to rule out uncontrolled production of parathyroid hormone from, for example, a parathyroid adenoma. There is nothing to suggest that this is the likely reason in this clinical context. There is no indication for measuring the serum aluminium, which is normally only measured in patients with suspected exposure to toxic levels of aluminium in drinking water.

---

2 D Intravenous fluids.

The patient has evidence of dehydration in that he has been reluctant to drink, has a high serum sodium and high serum urea, with a creatinine level within the normal range. In patients prone to hypercalcaemia because of malignant deposits in bone, dehydration is an important exacerbating factor. Therefore, in the first instance it would be most sensible to ensure that the patient is well hydrated with intravenous fluids. Intravenous pamidronate can be used in subjects with symptomatic hypercalcaemia associated with malignancy, though there is no reason to use that approach as a first-line management in this patient. Calcitonin does reduce the serum calcium; however, in the case of malignant hypercalcemia, substantial doses and sustained treatment would be required and is likely to be associated with unacceptable side-effects. Therefore it is not a reasonable option in these circumstances. The patient is already probably dehydrated so intravenous frusemide would not be appropriate, though in a fully hydrated patient, frusemide can help to reduce the serum calcium level in a hypercalcaemic individual. Strontium ranelate would not be expected to have any effect on the serum calcium concentration.

3 This patient has a normachromic anaemia that in this context is likely to be due to suppression of erythropoesis from direct infiltration of bone marrow by malignant deposits from his probable carcinoma of the prostate. There may also be an associated anaemia of chronic disease through indirect suppression of erythropoesis in the context of extensive malignancy.

4 Management of a patient with probable carcinoma of the prostate and extensive bony metastatic disease should be conducted in collaboration with an urologist. It is likely that histological confirmation would be obtained by prostatic biopsy. The PSA would be expected to be high or very high under these circumstances. The extent of the metastatic disease can be assessed further by performing an isotope bone scan.

Tutorial

Carcinoma of the prostate is common and is the second most frequently diagnosed malignant disease in men in the UK. It is usually a slow-growing malignancy and only about 25% of patients in whom the diagnosis is made die as a direct result of the disease. However, a substantial proportion of the patients will require treatment, largely aimed an ameliorating painful symptoms and lower urinary tract obstruction. The peak age band for presentation is 65–85 years. Most patients have well-differentiated adenocarcinomas with a relatively low propensity for metastases. However, it is thought that at least 50% of patients have some degree of metastatic disease once they become symptomatic. Treatment options, which should always be discussed with the urologist, include radical approaches such as combined prostatectomy and radical radiotherapy at one end of the spectrum, through to a wait-and-see policy centred around treating symptoms and problems if and when they arise. A large proportion of patients are able to have their prostatic carcinoma suppressed for long periods with hormonal treatments that deplete androgens, such as goserelin (orchidectomy has a similar effect), or that block androgen effects on the malignant cell line, for example cyproterone. PSA can be used for screening, though it gives no indication of the level of aggressiveness of the underlying tumour.

Patient 42

An 85-year-old woman was admitted urgently to hospital after a fall caused by a loss of balance on an uneven pavement. She was found to have a fractured left neck of femur that was treated the next day by insertion of an Austin Moore hemiarthroplasty. On the first post-operative day she started to have episodes of urinary incontinence, characterized by an urgent need to pass urine followed within less than a minute by the incontinent passage of a large volume of urine. On closer questioning it was found that she had experienced urgency of micturition of gradually increasing severity for about 1 year, though no incontinence had occurred. She had no other significant past medical history, though her daughter reported that her mother had become increasingly forgetful over the preceding 2 years or so. She was taking no medication. On examination, she was afebrile and had a clean operation scar. Her MMSE score was 19/30. Pulse was 76 bpm regular, BP 145/85 mmHg, heart sounds normal, respiratory rate 12 per minute, and auscultation of the chest was normal. Abdominal examination, including a per rectal examination, was normal. Visual inspection of the perineum revealed no obvious abnormalities other than a mild degree of atrophy of the external genitalia. On examination of her CNS there was generalized mild hyper-reflexia but no focal or lateralizing signs. Her gait was slightly short-stepping, though gait analysis was hampered by the recent surgery. She had exaggerated body sway in the standing position with her eyes open and closed. Bedside urine analysis showed a trace of protein but was otherwise normal.

Chest radiograph and ECG were normal. A postmicturition residual bladder volume, measured by ultrasound scan, was 70 ml.

Investigations (normal range)

Haemoglobin 12.7 g/L (11.5–16.5)
Total white cell count 4.8×10^9/L (4–11)
Serum urea 8.1 mmol/L (2.5–7.5)
Serum creatinine 84 µmol/L (60–110)
Serum sodium 140 mmol/L (137–144)
Serum potassium 3.9 mmol/L (3.5–4.9)
Plasma free thyroxine 18 pmol/L (10–22)

---

1 The most likely cause of her urinary incontinence is:
   A Constipation with faecal impaction.
   B Chronic retention of urine with overflow incontinence.
   C Detrusor-sphincter dysynergia.
   D Uninhibited neurogenic incontinence.
   E Partial uterine prolapse.

---

2 Outline the most important differential diagnoses for her neurological state.

---

3 The most important aspect of her treatment to try to regain continence is:
   A Insertion of a urinary catheter.
   B A course of broad-spectrum antibiotics.
   C Physiotherapy to restore independent walking.
   D Insertion of a ring pessary.
   E Fluid restriction.

---

4 Discuss potential drug therapies that might be of some help in the management of this patient's incontinence.

Patient 42 Answers

---
1 D Uninhibited neurogenic incontinence.

The description of the pattern of incontinence in this patient is typical of uninhibited micturition. This is the commonest pattern of incontinence in elderly patients and is caused by damage to central (mainly midbrain and frontal lobe) inhibitory centres by a wide range of brain pathologies including cerebrovascular disease, Alzheimer's disease, and other forms of dementia. The patient loses the ability to send inhibitory signals to the reflex mechanisms in the lower spinal cord. Consequently, the patient is unable to maintain high sphincteric tone and detrusor relaxation; the consequent detrusor contraction is then felt as an urgent need to pass urine and, as the condition progresses, urge incontinence. In the patient described, this is supported by the preadmission description of urgency of micturition, the gradual deterioration in that symptom, and the associated problems with short-term memory and a low MMSE score. Furthermore, there were no symptoms or physical signs of other contributing pathology. In this patient the actual incontinence has been precipitated by the reduced mobility consequent upon her fractured hip.

Constipation with faecal impaction is an important cause of both urinary incontinence (through direct pressure on the bladder and distortion of the urinary outflow tract) and retention of urine (particularly in elderly men). However, the patient described did not have faeces in the rectum or palpable faeces on examination of the abdomen. Patients with chronic retention of urine with overflow usually have a palpable bladder and would have a very large residual postmicturition volume detectable by ultrasonic bladder scanning. Furthermore, the pattern of the incontinence in such patients tends to be of frequent dribbling incontinence with small volumes voided and there is often a stress incontinence component manifested by leakage of urine on coughing, straining, or assuming the upright position. Detrusor-sphincter dysynergia is a relatively uncommon condition in which detrusor contraction is not coordinated with sphincter relaxation. The main symptom is painful micturition. Patients with uterine prolapse, particularly of minor degree, are often not incontinent of urine. If there is incontinence it is usually of the stress incontinence pattern with leakage of small volumes whenever there is a rise in intra-abdominal pressure.

2 The patient's neurological state consists of a history of failing memory, a moderately reduced MMSE score, mild hyper-reflexia, increased postural sway, and cognitive impairment. The most likely cause of this combination is cerebrovascular disease, though some patients with Alzheimer's disease would present with a virtually identical clinical picture. Other dementias should also be considered. Communicating hydrocephalus (sometimes called NPH) is an important cause of urinary incontinence and cognitive impairment. The time course of the symptoms is usually shorter than that described for this patient, though there is considerable variation. Though the condition is relatively rare, it is important to make the diagnosis because of the potential benefit of a shunt to reduce intracerebral pressure. CT scanning is an important investigation in this context, particularly to rule out NPH and other potentially treatable conditions such as intracerebral tumours. A CT scan would be expected, in the patient described, to show evidence of cerebrovascular disease in the form of atrophy, reduced grey–white matter differentiation, and possibly multiple infarcts.

---
3 C Physiotherapy to restore independent walking.

This patient has become incontinent because of her abruptly reduced mobility. Prior to admission she had urgency of micturition but was continent. Therefore, the most fruitful focus of treatment would be to regain mobility as quickly as possible with physiotherapy. There is no indication for passing a urinary catheter in this patient, though that option can be kept in reserve if the patient finds the flooding incontinence intolerable and expresses a preference for a catheter or if catheterization is required to help maintain skin integrity. Similarly, as there is no evidence of infection, there is nothing to be gained by giving antibiotics and the unnecessary use of antibiotics can result in serious antibiotic-associated complications. A ring pessary can sometimes help patients with uterine prolapse with stress incontinence but would not be expected to have any effect in the condition described in this case. There is no place for routine fluid restriction. If elderly patients are fluid-restricted in this context, they easily become dehydrated and all that is gained is that the episodes of flooding incontinence would be slightly less frequent. Occasionally, restriction of fluids in the evening can help to reduce the frequency of nocturnal micturition and can then be part of an overall management plan for the patient. Such an option requires a patient who is fully *compos mentis* or fully supervised to be effective and to avoid dehydration.

4 Patients with unininhibited neurogenic micturition can be helped with antimuscarinic agents such as oxybutynin and tolterodine. However, simply prescribing these drugs is not likely to result in a satisfactory outcome. They reduce detrusor tone and thereby increase the volume at which the urgent need to pass urine is felt. If combined with a regular toileting regimen and attempts to improve mobility, such drugs can be part of an overall management package for a patient with uninhibited detrusor contractions.

Antimuscarinic drugs should be used cautiously in elderly patients as they may precipitate retention of urine (particularly in elderly men with prostatic hypertrophy) and can have unwanted effects in patients with autonomic impairment. In particular, they tend to worsen postural hypotension and tend to be arrhythmogenic. Such drugs should be avoided in patients with closed angle glaucoma. Patients who have well-preserved cognitive function or are supervised, yet still have a tendency to nocturnal frequency of urine, can sometimes be helped by using desmopressin (a vasopressin analogue) at night. This treatment requires close supervision and some patients tend to retain excess water and become hyponatraemic.

Patient 43

An 81-year-old man was brought to hospital urgently with severe shortness of breath of about 10 hours duration. He was previously well apart from a history of hypertension and stable mild chronic renal failure. He had signs of cardiac failure and his pulse was 120 bpm and irregularly irregular. His body weight was 60 kg.

An ECG showed atrial fibrillation with a ventricular rate of 125 per minute but no evidence of acute MI. A chest radiograph showed signs of early pulmonary oedema. An urgent echocardiogram showed moderate reduction in left ventricular contractility and a left atrial diameter of 4.8 cm (normal <3.8 cm). Review of his previous blood tests showed that his serum creatinine had been at 160, 175 and 168 µmol/L at 2-monthly intervals over the previous 6 months. There was a good response to oxygen therapy and intravenous frusemide with a rapid resolution of his dyspnoea. A decision was made to control his atrial fibrillation with oral digoxin loading on the grounds that he was unlikely to be easily converted to sinus rhythm.

Investigations (normal range)

Haemoglobin 14.7 g/dL (13–18)
Total white cell count 6.8 × 10⁹/L (4–11)
Serum urea 20 mmol/L (2.5–7.5)
Serum creatinine 118 µmol (60–110)
Serum sodium 142 mmol/L (137–144)
Serum potassium 4.9 mmol/L (3.5–4.9)
Serum CK 85 U/L (24–195)
Serum troponin T undetectable
Serum ALT 55 U/L (5–35)
Serum alkaline phosphatase 110 U/L (45–105)
Serum total bilirubin 29 µmol/L (1–22)
Oxygen saturation on room air 93%

1 The loading dose of digoxin is determined by:
   A Estimated GFR.
   B Estimated lean body mass.
   C The patient's age.
   D The patient's heart rate.
   E Liver reserve function.

2 For the patient described in this case, the digoxin total loading dose is about:
   A 100 µg.
   B 1000 µg.
   C 2000 µg.
   D 3000 µg.
   E 4000 µg.

3 The maintenance dose for digoxin is mainly dependent upon:
   A The patient's age.
   B The estimated lean body mass.
   C The estimated GFR.
   D Serum urea concentration.
   E Serum potassium concentration.

4 The main reason for choosing digoxin to control the ventricular rate in this patient is:
   A His age.
   B The presence of chronic renal failure.
   C His impaired liver function.
   D The dilated left atrium.
   E The presentation with cardiac failure.

Patient 43 Answers

> **1 B** Estimated lean body mass.

Digoxin binds to muscle cells so the loading dose to achieve a therapeutic level is determined mainly by the patient's lean body mass. The patient's age only affects the loading dose insofar as lean body mass falls with age, and that does need to be taken into account to a certain extent. The heart rate response to dosing is important and can be a guide to the total loading dose if loading is conducted over several days rather than rapidly. Nevertheless, the factor that determines the loading dose required to achieve rate control remains closely related to lean body mass. Liver reserve function is not important in this context because digoxin is largely excreted renally. However, the GFR, even if substantially reduced, does not influence the total initial dose required to achieve therapeutic tissue concentrations.

> **2 B** 1000 μg.

For an elderly man with a body weight of 60 kg the closest option would be 1000 μg as the estimated total loading dose. A dose of 100 μg would certainly be ineffective and the patient of this size would probably reach a toxic level of serum digoxin if 2000 μg or more were given in less than 24 hours.

> **3 C** The estimated GFR.

Because digoxin is excreted mainly through renal filtration, the main determinant of the maintenance dose is the patient's GFR. This can be estimated from the patient's serum creatinine and age, adjusting for race and sex. However, in practical terms precise estimation or measurement is not required. More usually in clinical practice the maintenance dose of digoxin is reduced in older patients, particularly if they have some evidence of renal impairment. In patients with more substantial degrees of renal impairment, it would be necessary to monitor the serum digoxin level. The patient's age is a relevant factor because it influences GFR (GFR falls with age). Lean body mass is of less importance in determining the maintenance dose required. The serum urea concentration is not an accurate means of estimating renal function and the serum potassium is only important in that patients who are hypokalaemic will be disproportionately sensitive to the effects of digoxin and *vice versa* for patients who are hyperkalaemic. Therefore,

serum potassium concentration needs to be taken into account when assessing the efficacy or side-effects of digoxin. In clinical practice the essential step would be to try to achieve a normokalaemic state in patients prescribed digoxin.

> **4 D** The dilated left atrium.

In this patient the main reason for choosing digoxin to control the ventricular rate was the dilated left atrium. Such patients are more likely to remain in sustained or paroxysmal atrial fibrillation, so choosing a drug that is aimed at promoting and maintaining sinus rhythm, such as amiodarone or sotalol is less likely to be effective when the left atrium is dilated. When there is a clear-cut precipitating cause of atrial fibrillation and the left atrial diameter is within or close to the normal range, an attempt should be made to re-establish sinus rhythm. The haemodynamic advantage of a higher cardiac output in sinus rhythm can make a substantial difference to the exercise tolerance of older patients. Age in itself would not determine the choice of medication in this case. The presence of chronic renal failure would determine the maintenance dose but not the choice of digoxin in these circumstances. In this patient's case, the chronic renal failure was not sufficiently severe to make digoxin an impractical choice. Impaired liver function in this patient was almost certainly due to hepatic congestion associated with the episode of acute heart failure, but in any case would not be a factor in choosing digoxin in the patient described. The presence of heart failure is a secondary reason for using digoxin in this context as there is some evidence that the positive inotropic effect of digoxin is beneficial. However, that is a relatively minor consideration because the improvement in cardiac dynamics with treatment of digoxin in the patient described would be mainly due to the improved cardiac output consequent upon better control of the ventricular response rate.

Patient 44

A 65-year-old man presented with a right hemiparesis. His BP on admission was 170/90 mmHg. The CT scanner broke down and it was not be possible to perform a scan for at least another 48 hours.

1 What is the best course of action?
   A Start warfarin.
   B Wait for a CT scan to be available.
   C Start clopidogrel.
   D Transfer to another hospital.
   E Start aspirin.

Patient 45

A 75-year-old man was brought to the Accident and Emergency Department after being found on the floor by his daughter. Physical examination revealed a left homonymous hemianopia and a left hemiparesis affecting both upper and lower limbs. He was noted to have left-sided sensory inattention and dysphasia.
A CT head scan (**45**) was performed.

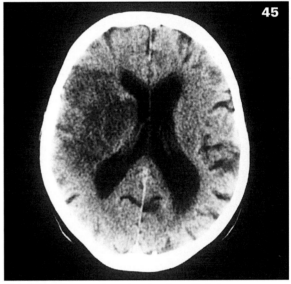

45 CT head scan taken shortly after admission.

1 Which statement best describes the appearance of the scan?
   A Cerebral infarct in the middle cerebral artery territory without midline shift.
   B Cerebral infarct in the anterior cerebral artery without midline shift.
   C Cerebral infarct in the middle cerebral artery territory with midline shift.
   D Glioblastoma multiforme causing midline shift.
   E Cerebral infarct in the anterior cerebral artery with midline shift.

2 How would you classify this patient's stroke?
   A LACI.
   B TIA.
   C TACI.
   D PACI.
   E POCI.

3 What is the likelihood of the patient being alive and independent at 1 year?
   A Less than 10%.
   B 10–20%.
   C 20–30%.
   D 30–40%.
   E 40–50%.

Patient 44 Answer

> **1 E** Start aspirin.

One systematic review of patients with an ischaemic stroke, confirmed by CT scan, found that aspirin compared to placebo within 48 hours significantly reduced death and dependency at 6 months and increased the number of people making a complete recovery. There is indirect evidence that starting aspirin should not be delayed if a scanner is not available within 48 hours. Two large randomized controlled trials found no detrimental effect of aspirin compared to placebo in patients subsequently found to have a haemorrhagic stroke.

Patient 45 Answers

> **1 C** Cerebral infarct in the middle cerebral artery territory with midline shift.

The scan shows a cerebral infarct in the territory of the middle cerebral artery. There is midline shift visible.

> **2 C** TACI.

In 1991 Bamford *et al.* devised a method of classifying strokes according to their clinical presentation. The classification (*Table 45a*) enables clinicians to determine the prognosis and possible aetiology of the stroke. A TACI and a PACI are most likely to be due to cerebral embolism, while a POCI and a LACI are more likely to be due to thrombosis *in situ*.

> **3 A** Less than 10%.

The classification allows the clinician to advise on the likely prognosis after the stroke (*Table 45b*).

Table 45a *Bamford classification of stroke*

Subtype	Clinical features
TACI	• Weakness &/or sensory deficit of at least 2 areas of face, arm, or leg • Homonymous hemianopia • New disturbance of higher cerebral function such as dysphasia or a visuospatial disorder
PACI	• 2 of the 3 components of a TACI
POCI	• Definite signs of brainstem or cerebellar disturbance, or • Isolated homonymous hemianopia
LACI	• Pure motor stroke • Pure sensory stroke • Pure sensorimotor stroke • Ataxic hemiparesis

Table 45b *Prognosis for stroke subtypes*

Subtype	Alive and independent at 1 year (%)	Alive but dependent at 1 year (%)	Annual risk of recurrent strokes (%)
TACI	4	36	6
PACI	55	29	17 (mostly early risk)
POCI	62	19	20 (continuing risk)
LACI	60	28	9

Patient 46

A 75-year-old woman presented with a long-standing history of abdominal pain and constipation. A barium enema was performed. Figure **46** shows a late film from that procedure.

1 What is the most likely cause of her abdominal pain?
 A Irritable bowel syndrome.
 B Diverticular disease.
 C Carcinoma of the colon.
 D Laxative abuse.
 E Sigmoid volvulus.

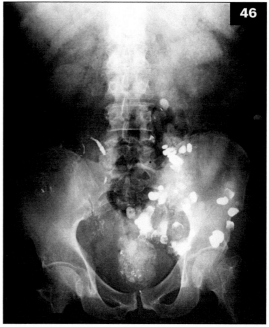

46 Barium enema – late film.

Patient 47

A 75-year-old man presented with a history of rectal bleeding. Physical examination was unremarkable. His haemoglobin was 10.1g/dL (13–18) with a MCV of 75 fL (80–96). His barium enema is shown in Figure **47**.

1 What is the most likely diagnosis?
 A Carcinoma of the colon.
 B Ulcerative colitis.
 C Ischaemic colitis.
 D Pneumatosis coli.
 E Volvulus.

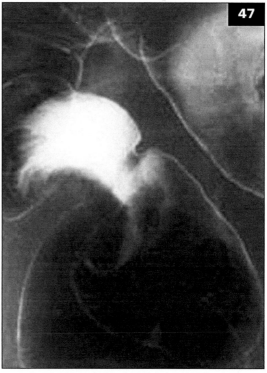

47 Detail from double contrast barium enema.

Patient 46 Answer

> **1 B** Diverticular disease.

The radiograph is a delayed abdominal image following a barium enema. The large white flecks of barium seen predominantly to the left of the abdomen are due to barium trapped within diverticula. Diverticular disease can occur in the presence of other pathology such as carcinoma of the colon, but diverticular disease is not a risk factor for developing carcinoma of the colon. Irritable bowel syndrome, laxative abuse, and a sigmoid volvulus can all cause abdominal pain but the radiograph suggests a more plausible diagnosis.

Tutorial

Diverticular disease is primarily a disease of industrialized western societies. Diet may influence the prevalence. Among Asians, diverticular disease has a right-sided predominance. The incidence increases with age and one third of the general UK population develops some degree of diverticulosis by the age of 45 years, and two thirds by 85 years. It is equally common in men and women. Diverticular disease can involve any part of the GI tract. The lesions are herniations of the mucosa and submucosa or the entire wall thickness through the muscularis, as seen in congenital diverticula. The sigmoid is the most commonly affected segment (95–98%); however the descending, ascending, and transverse colon as well as the jejunum, ileum, and duodenum can also be involved. The exact aetiology of this disease is unknown. It is believed that high intraluminal pressure and a weak colonic wall at the sites of nutrient vessel penetration into the muscularis leads to herniation and diverticula formation. The condition can also be caused by abnormal colonic motility, defective muscular structure, defects in collagen consistency (i.e. increased cross-linking of collagen), and ageing.

Diverticulitis and lower GI bleeding secondary to diverticulosis are the main complications of clinical importance to emergency physicians. Acute diverticulitis results from the inspissation of faecal material in the neck of the diverticulum and resultant bacterial replication. It may be complicated by abscess formation or peridiverticular inflammation initiated by the rupture of a microscopic mucosal abscess into the mesentery. This may progress, fistulize, obstruct, or spontaneously resolve. Lower GI bleeding from diverticulosis results from rupture of the small blood vessels that are stretched while coursing over the dome of the diverticula. Mortality and morbidity are related to complications of diverticulosis. These occur in 10–20% of patients with diverticulosis during their lifetime.

Patient 47 Answer

> **1 A** Carcinoma of the colon.

The barium enema shows a classsic 'apple core' appearance in the region of the descending colon. This is suggestive of carcinoma of the colon.

Tutorial

Carcinoma of the bowel is one of the commonest malignant tumours. It is commoner in the western world and is thought to be related to a diet low in fibre.

Patient 48

A 74-year-old woman presented with an iron deficiency anaemia. Figure **48** is taken from the patient's transverse colon.

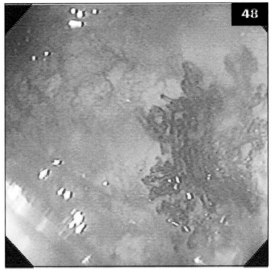

48 Appearance of the colonic mucosa.

1 What is the most likely cause of her anaemia?
   A Hereditary haemorrhagic telangectasia.
   B Angiodysplasia.
   C Varices.
   D Ulcerative colitis.
   E Mesenteric ischaemia.

Patient 49

An 86-year-old man complained of a 2-week history of dysphagia to solids. His chest radiograph and 'barium' swallow are shown (**49a**, **49b**).

1 What is the most likely cause of his symptoms?
   A Metastatic carcinoma of the lung.
   B Oesophageal varices.
   C Oesophageal candidiasis.
   D Cervical osteophytic dysphagia.
   E Oesophageal carcinoma.

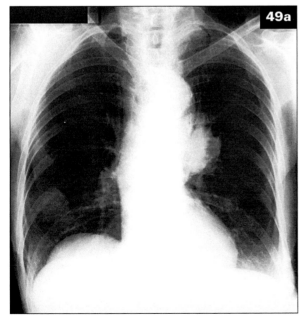

49a Chest radiograph of patient presenting with dysphagia.

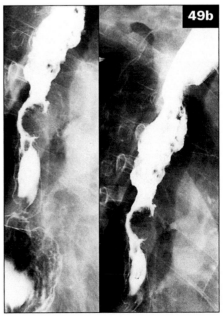

49b 'Barium' swallow from the same patient.

Patient 48 Answer

1 B Angiodysplasia.

The appearance is typical of intestinal angiodysplasia.

Tutorial

Angiodysplasia occurs mostly in the colon but can also occur in other parts of the bowel such as the stomach. It is a condition of stretching and dilatation of fragile blood vessels that results in occasional blood loss. It is mostly associated with ageing and is due to degeneration of blood vessels. It is thought to develop as a result of the rhythmic contractions of the colon causing stretching of blood vessels and development of small arterio-venous fistulae leading to the angiodysplasia. It is a common cause of bleeding, present in about 5% of bleeders and 3% of persons without overt blood loss.

It is diagnosed at colonoscopy or mesenteric angiography. The latter gives a positive result during periods of active bleeding. Treatment depends on the rate of bleeding. In 90% of cases bleeding stops spontaneously. Some require cautery or resection of a segment of bowel.

Patient 49 Answer

1 A Metastatic carcinoma of the lung.

The barium swallow (**49b**) shows multiple lesions causing extrinsic compression of the oesophagus at multiple levels. The chest radiograph shows an enlarged left hilum indicating a carcinoma of the bronchus. The dysphagia is therefore most likely to be due to metastatic carcinoma of the lung.

Tutorial

Dysphagia can occur because of pathology in the mouth, pharynx, or oesophagus. The causes of dysphagia can be divided into mechanical or neuromuscular causes. *Table 49* lists possible causes.

Table 49 *Causes of dysphagia*

Mechanical	Neuromuscular
• Malignancy (pharynx, oesophagus, stomach)	• Achalasia
• Infection (oesophageal Candida, CMV)	• Myasthenia gravis
• Reflux oesophagitis	• Diffuse oesophageal spasm
• Benign stricture (oesophagus, peptic)	• Scleroderma (CREST)
• Intraluminal foreign body	• Bulbar palsy
• Pharyngeal pouch	• Pseudobulbar palsy
• Extrinsic compression (lung cancer, mediastinal lymph nodes, retrosternal goitre, aortic aneurysm, left atrial enlargement, cervical osteophytes)	• Syringobulbia
	• Chagas disease

Patient 50

An 81-year-old woman was admitted to hospital with foul smelling diarrhoea. There was blood in the stools. She had had a chest infection 2 weeks previously for which she had just completed a course of cefaclor. *Clostridium difficile* was suspected.

---

1 Which of these tests would be most useful in confirming the diagnosis?
  A Blood culture.
  B CRP.
  C Raised IgM antibodies.
  D Stool microscopy.
  E Sigmoidoscopy and biopsy.

Patient 51

An 84-year-old independent woman who lived on her own complained of a sensation of fullness on eating small amounts of food. She had a previous history of peptic ulceration. She claimed that solid food stuck in the middle of her chest. Very often she vomited undigested food. Her 'barium' swallow is shown below (**51**).

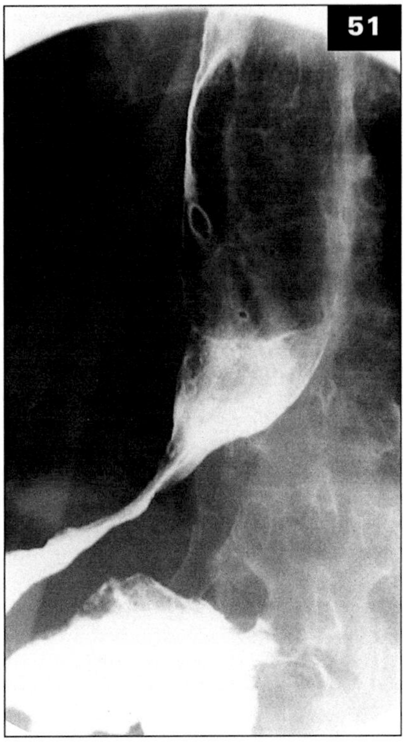

51 'Barium' swallow of a patient presenting with dysphagia.

---

1 What will be the most appropriate course of action?
  A Perform an OGD with dilatation of the stricture.
  B Inform the patient she has cancer and refer her for palliative care.
  C Inform the patient she has cancer and refer her for surgery.
  D Inform the patient she has cancer and refer her for radiotherapy.
  E Perform an OGD and start omeprazole.

Patient 50 Answer

1 E Sigmoidoscopy and biopsy.

The patient's history is very suggestive of *Clostridium difficile* diarrhoea. The best way to diagnose *C. difficile* is isolation of the organism from the stool or detection of toxin in the stool. Sigmoidoscopy and biopsy can be of value in diagnosing *C. difficile* complicated by pseudo-membraneous colitis. *C. difficile* infection is not a bacteraemic infection; therefore, blood cultures are of no use in obtaining a diagnosis. Similarly antibody tests and stool microscopy are of no value in this context. Any rise in C-reactive protein would be nonspecific and therefore not helpful.

Tutorial

C. difficile is a Gram-positive, anaerobic, spore-forming bacillus that is responsible for the development of antibiotic-associated diarrhoea and colitis. It is called *difficile* (difficult) because it grows slowly and is hard to culture. The infection commonly manifests as mild-to-moderate diarrhoea with abdominal cramping and a low-grade fever. Pseudo-membranes, adherent yellowish-white plaques on the intestinal mucosa, are occasionally observed. In rare cases, patients with *C. difficile* infection can present with an acute abdomen and fulminant life-threatening colitis. The diagnosis of colitis should be suspected in any patient with diarrhoea who has received antibiotics within the previous 2 months and/or when diarrhoea occurs 72 hours or more after hospitalization.

C. difficile colitis results from a disturbance of the normal bacterial flora of the colon, colonization by and overgrowth of *C. difficile*, and release of toxins (toxin A is an enterotoxin, and toxin B is a cytotoxin) that bind to the mucosa causing mucosal inflammation and damage. Antibiotic therapy is the key factor that alters the colonic flora and allows the population of *C. difficile* to rise unchecked in the lumen. Hospitalized patients are at highest risk of the infection. *C. difficile* is present in 2–3% of healthy adults. Approximately 20% of individuals who are hospitalized acquire the organism, and more than 30% of these patients develop diarrhoea. Thus, *C. difficile* colitis is currently one of the most common nosocomial infections. Colonization occurs by the faecal–oral route. *C. difficile* forms heat-resistant spores that can persist in the environment for several months to years. Outbreaks occur in hospitals and other outpatient facilities where contamination with spores is prevalent. Normal gut flora resists colonization and overgrowth with *C. difficile* while antibiotic use, which suppresses the normal flora, allows proliferation.

C. difficile colitis is therefore almost exclusively associated with antibiotic usage (*Table 50*). Even brief exposure to any single antibiotic can cause the condition. A prolonged antibiotic course or the use of two or more antibiotics increases the risk of disease. Even antibiotics traditionally used to treat *C. difficile* colitis have been shown to cause the disease.

Treatment of asymptomatic carriers is not recommended as most patients with *C. difficile* colitis recover without specific therapy. However, symptoms may be prolonged and debilitating. Reports that focus on patients who are more seriously ill indicate mortality rates of 10–30%. The decision to treat the infection and the choice of therapy depends on the severity of the disease. Cessation of the causative antibiotic is essential when possible, and this can be sufficient to control mild disease. This conservative approach allows for reconstitution of the normal colonic microflora and markedly reduces the risk of relapse. Patients with more severe diarrhoea or colitis should receive antibiotic therapy directed at *C. difficile*. More than 95% of patients respond to 10 days of treatment with vancomycin (oral) or metronidazole (oral or intravenous). Symptomatic improvement can be expected within 2–3 days. The oral administration of these medications is the preferred route because *C. difficile* remains within the colonic lumen without invading the colonic mucosa. Vancomycin is poorly absorbed in the intestinal tract, thereby promoting high concentrations within the intestinal lumen while significantly reducing the prevalence of adverse systemic effects. Metronidazole, despite the incidence of systemic adverse effects and isolation of metronidazole-resistant strains of the organism, is the drug of first choice because of its lower cost. There is also evidence that it is more effective than vancomycin. For patients who are unable to tolerate oral medication, intravenous metronidazole is effective. Excretion of the drug into bile and exudation from the inflamed colon results in bactericidal levels in faeces. Intravenous vancomycin is ineffective in this condition.

In general, relapse is common and occurs in 5–50% of cases. Relapse usually occurs 3 days to 3 weeks after treatment is discontinued. Relapse may occur due to failure to eradicate the organism or reinfection from the environment. Fulminant colitis and toxic megacolon often require surgical treatment.

Table 50 *Risk factors for Clostridium difficile infection*

- Cephalosporins (especially 2nd and 3rd generation)
- Ampicillin/amoxicillin and clindamycin
- Less commonly implicated antibiotics are the macrolides (i.e. erythromycin, clarithromycin, azithromycin) and other penicillins
- Agents occasionally implicated include aminoglycosides, fluoroquinolones, metronidazole, chloramphenicol, tetracycline, imipenem, and meropenem
- Advanced age (>60 years)
- Contact with infected persons

Rarer associations
- Antineoplastic agents, principally methotrexate
- Haemolytic–uraemic syndrome
- Malignancies
- Intestinal ischaemia
- Renal failure
- Necrotizing enterocolitis
- Hirschsprung's disease
- Inflammatory bowel disease

Patient 51 Answer

1 A Perform an OGD with dilatation of the stricture.

This patient has a stricture at the lower end of the oesophagus. The radiological features suggest that this is a benign stricture. There is a grossly dilated oesophagus above a smoothly constricted section of the oesophagus.

The best course of action would be to perform a gastroscopy with dilatation of the stricture, if the patient's physical condition allows it. This will also give the opportunity of taking a biopsy to confirm the benign nature of the stricture. The most likely aetiology of the stricture is fibrosis secondary to reflux oesophagitis, so starting a proton pump inhibitor would be important to suppress acid production. However, at this stage that would be insufficient to relieve this patient's symptoms.

Patient 52

A 70-year-old woman was referred for investigation of weight loss. She gave a history of long-standing abdominal distension, pain, and foul smelling diarrhoea. She had returned to the UK having spent several years working in Africa. Physical examination revealed a BMI of 15 kg/m². Her plain abdominal radiograph is shown (**52**).

Investigations (normal range)

Haemoglobin 9.2 g/dL (11.5–16.5)
Haematocrit 0.45 (0.36–0.47)
MCV 103 fL (80–96)
MCH 22 pg (28–32)
Total leukocyte count 9.4 × 10⁹/L (4-11)
Platelets 130 × 10⁹/L (150–400)
INR 1.4
Serum amylase 150 U/L (60–180)

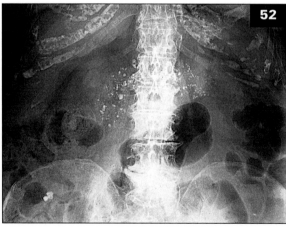

52 Plain abdominal radiograph in a patient presenting with weight loss.

1 What is the likely cause of her symptoms?
  A Ulcerative colitis.
  B Ischaemic colitis.
  C Tropical sprue.
  D Coeliac disease.
  E Pancreatitis.

2 Which is the *least* useful in managing this patient?
  A HbA1C
  B Serum CA 125.
  C Serum CA 19-9.
  D ERCP.
  E Fat-soluble vitamin supplements.

Patient 52 Answer

1 E Pancreatitis.

The plain abdominal radiograph shows calcification throughout the pancreas particularly around the area of the head of pancreas. This makes the diagnosis of chronic calcific pancreatitis the most likely. Amylase levels are variable and not necessarily elevated. Elevated amylase readings are a reflection of ongoing inflammation.

2 B Serum CA 125.

This patient presented with a history suggestive of malabsorbtion (causes of malabsorbtion are shown in *Table 52*). The radiological findings suggest pancreatitis as the cause of her symptoms. Serum CA 125 is a tumour marker raised in a variety of ovarian diseases including ovarian cancer and so is not relevant to the investigation of this case. CA 19-9 is raised in cancers of the digestive tract particularly pancreatic cancer. The test cannot be recommended for cancer screening; however, it can be useful in monitoring disease. It might be useful for investigating this woman, as cancer of the pancreas is one of the main possible diagnoses to be considered. Two to four percent of all American patients with pancreatic calcification have coexisting pancreatic carcinoma. It appears that alcoholism and chronic pancreatitis in some way predispose to development of pancreatic malignancy. When calcification occurs together with pancreatic cancer, it usually indicates pre-existing pancreatitis. Occasionally it is present only proximal to a tumour that has occluded the pancreatic duct and these patients may not have had any previous pancreatitis.

Patients with pancreatitis very often develop diabetes and an HbA1C is an important investigation to perform. An ERCP is important in establishing a diagnosis. This woman has steatorrhoea and evidence of vitamin K deficiency. Fat-soluble vitamin supplements are an important part in her management. She is also likely to benefit from pancreatic enzyme supplements.

Table 52 *Differential diagnosis of malabsorption*

Site	Pathology
Stomach	• Postgastrectomy • Pernicious anaemia • Zollinger Ellison syndrome
Pancreas	• Pancreatitis • Carcinoma of the pancreas • Cystic fibrosis
Hepatobiliary	• Obstruction • Cholestasis
Small intestine	• Coeliac disease • Crohn's disease • Lymphoma • Fistulae and blind loops • Infections, bacterial overgrowth/parasites • Radiation • Whipple's disease • Drugs, e.g. cholestyramine • Surgery and removal of small bowel

Tutorial

Pancreatic calcification may occur in a number of conditions. About 90% of the patients with calcification have alcoholic pancreatitis. Such patients often give a history of long-standing alcoholism with frequent severe abdominal pain.

Hereditary pancreatitis may be suspected when large, rounded pancreatic calculi are shown. A positive family history is the most important diagnostic element in such cases. If associated with nephrocalcinosis, hyperparathyroidism should be suspected.

Some patients with cystic fibrosis and diabetes mellitus also have pancreatic calcification. In underdeveloped nations, pancreatic calcification is frequently observed in association with protein malnutrition. Tumour calcification may occur in cystadenoma , cystadenocarcinoma, and cavernous lymphangioma.

Occasional instances of pancreatic calcification occur in patients without any clinical evidence of pancreatic disease. These patients usually have nonspecific pancreatic ductal stenosis with calculi forming beyond the site of obstruction. Idiopathic senile chronic pancreatitis appears to be a special subtype of nonalcoholic chronic pancreatitis. The main clinical features are onset after the age of 50 years, higher prevalence in men, a painless clinical course, weight loss associated with diarrhoea (steatorrhoea) or diabetes mellitus, and pancreatic calcific deposits. It is thought to have an autoimmune aetiology.

Patient 53

A 72-year-old man presented with headaches. Physical examination showed a BP of 180/85 mmHg. He was referred for a 24 hour ambulatory BP recording (**53a**).

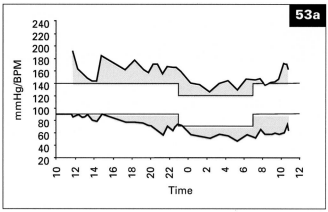

53a 24-hour BP recording.

1 What does the tracing show?
   A ISH.
   B Normal recording.
   C White coat hypertension.
   D Systo-diastolic hypertension.
   E Hypertensive nondipper.

Patient 54

A 79-year-old man of south Asian origin presented with shortness of breath, lower limb oedema, and ascites. His lateral chest radiograph is shown (**54**). He had a strongly positive tuberculin test although he had never been diagnosed as having TB.

54 Plain lateral chest radiograph.

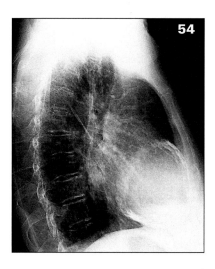

1 What is the most likely cause of his symptoms?
   A Acute pericarditis.
   B Pulmonary TB.
   C Miliary TB.
   D Chronic calcific pericarditis.
   E Chronic liver disease.

Patient 55

A 75-year-old retired dockyard worker with a long-standing history of hypertension presented with lower limb oedema. He denied any shortness of breath. He was taking amlodipine 5 mg and bendroflumethiazide 2.5 mg once daily. Physical examination revealed a BMI of 28 kg/m². His BP in clinic was 185/90 mmHg. An electrocardiogram showed sinus rhythm with left ventricular hypertrophy.

A chest radiograph showed upper lobe blood diversion and a cardiothoracic ratio of 18/30. An ultrasound scan of the kidneys was normal.

Investigations (normal range)

Serum sodium 145 mmol/L (137–144)
Serum potassium 4.0 mmol/L (3.5–4.9)
Serum urea 8.0 mmol/L (2.5–7.5)
Serum creatinine 145 µmol/L (60–110)

1 What was the best course of action?
   A Advise the patient to see his GP and make no changes yet.
   B Advise the patient to lose weight and monitor his lower limb oedema.
   C Advise weight loss and increase the dose of his amlodipine and diuretic.
   D Stop the amlodipine and change to an angiotensin II receptor antagonist.
   E Perform a 24 hour BP monitor and review.

Patient 53 Answer

---

1 A ISH.

This is an example of ISH. One can see that over a 24-hour period the diastolic BP is within the normal range while the systolic BP is raised. White coat hypertension is a condition where people have an elevated BP reading when measured in clinic but normal readings when the ambulatory method is used to record their BP at home.

The cardiovascular risk of these patients is much smaller than those with sustained hypertension. White coat hypertension needs to be distinguished from superimposed white coat 'effect' in which the BP recorded in clinic is higher than the average daytime reading which is nonetheless elevated above normal. Systo-diastolic hypertension refers to a rise in both systolic and diastolic readings. A hypertensive nondipper is when there is no drop in nocturnal BP.

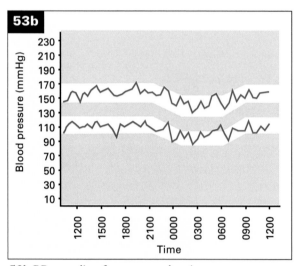

53b BP recording from a normal patient.

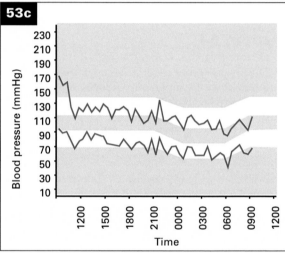

53c White coat hypertension. (Note the elevated readings at the beginning of the test when the equipment is being put on.)

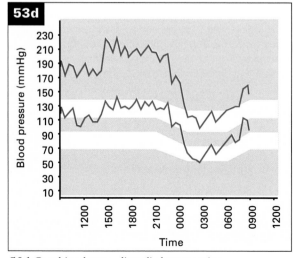

53d Combined systo-diastolic hypertension.

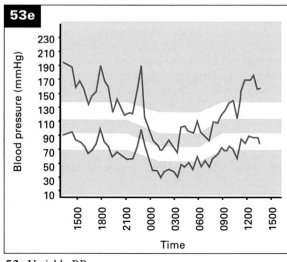

53e Variable BP.

Tutorial (Patient 53)

ISH is defined as a systolic BP ≥140 mmHg and a diastolic BP <90 mmHg. In the industrialized world systolic BP rises with age and is higher in men than in women until the age of 70 years. Diastolic BP rises with age until 60 years in men and 75 in women and falls thereafter. This leads to a state in which the pulse pressure (systolic minus diastolic BP) increases with age. These BP changes are sometimes referred to as being normal but are in fact the result of several pathological processes. In societies where the incidence of hypertension is low, BP does not rise with age. ISH is the commonest form of hypertension in old age. This is due to the excessive rise in systolic BP accompanied by a declining diastolic BP, probably largely the result of reduced compliance of large arteries.

Several studies have demonstrated an increased risk for cardiovascular and cerebrovascular diseases and death in patients with ISH. Untreated ISH leads to left ventricular hypertrophy that is associated with a poor cardiovascular prognosis.

Several trials of hypertension that included elderly patients above 60 years have shown benefit in treating elevated BP. Two studies, SHEP (systolic hypertension in elderly patients) and SYST-EUR (a Europe-wide study), showed that treating ISH (≥160 mmHg) reduced cardiovascular events.

24 hour BP monitoring is useful in assessing a patient's average BP reading if white coat hypertension is suspected, and to monitor the effect of treatment on patients on two or more antihypertensives. Figures **53b–53e** show a series of patterns commonly seen in elderly patients.

Patient 54 Answer

1 D Chronic calcific pericarditis.

His presentation is one suggesting constrictive pericarditis. The lateral chest radiograph (**54**) shows curvilinear calcification surrounding the heart. Calcification of the degree shown is associated with tuberculous pericarditis. It usually present as thick, amorphous calcification along the atrioventricular groove. This pattern is observed less commonly with other forms of pericarditis.

Pericarditis is seen in 1–2% of all cases of pulmonary TB. Extensive tuberculous pericarditis is rare in Anglo–Celtic populations. Of patients with pericardial calcification, 50–70% have constrictive pericarditis. The major subtypes of chronic pericarditis are chronic constrictive pericarditis and chronic effusive pericarditis.

Pericardial fibrosis or calcification is asymptomatic unless chronic constrictive pericarditis occurs. Symptoms and signs of peripheral venous congestion may appear along with an early diastolic sound, often best heard on inspiration (pericardial knock), due to abrupt slowing of diastolic ventricular filling by the rigid pericardium. Signs of chronic constrictive pericarditis differ from cardiac tamponade. The only early abnormalities may be elevated ventricular diastolic, atrial, pulmonary, and systemic venous pressures. Ventricular systolic function (ejection fraction) is usually preserved. Prolonged elevation of pulmonary venous pressure results in dyspnoea and orthopnoea. Systemic venous hypertension produces hypervolemia, engorgement of neck veins, pleural effusion (usually greater on the right side), hepatomegaly, ascites, and peripheral oedema. Pulsus paradoxus occurs in few cases of calcific pericarditis and is usually less severe than in tamponade.

Kussmaul's sign (swelling of the neck veins on inspiration, and referred to as venous paradox) is sometimes present, whereas it is usually absent in cardiac tamponade.

ECG changes are nonspecific. QRS voltage is usually low. T waves are usually nonspecifically abnormal. Atrial fibrillation (less commonly, atrial flutter) is present in about 25% of patients with constrictive pericarditis. Cardiac catheterization shows equalization of diastolic pressures in all four chambers, with a positive square root sign (pattern of ventricular diastolic pressure characteristic of constrictive pericarditis).

Chronic constrictive pericarditis may lead to effusive-constrictive pericarditis, in which the intracardiac pressure recordings are similar to those of cardiac tamponade but, after the pericardial fluid is removed, are similar to those of chronic constrictive pericarditis.

Tutorial

Calcification of the pericardium is usually preceded by pericarditis or trauma. It seldom follows rheumatic fever but among the more common known causes are:
- TB or other infections including viral agents (e.g. coxsackievirus, influenza A, influenza B) and histoplasmosis.
- Pericardial tumours, such as intrapericardial teratomas and pericardial cysts.
- Connective tissue disease including RA and SLE.
- Trauma causing a haemopericardium, including cardiac surgery.
- Uraemic pericarditis.

Patient 55 Answer

> **1 D** Stop the amlodipine and change to an angiotensin II receptor antagonist.

This patient's BP is high. He has evidence of end-organ damage and he needs effective treatment. It is well known that BP is often elevated in clinic, an effect known as white coat hypertension; however, it is not sufficient to attribute the patient's raised BP to this effect. The British Hypertension Society suggests an audit standard for BP control in clinic of 150/90 mmHg. While losing weight is an important recommendation, it is unlikely to be effective in controlling this patient's BP on its own. The combination of a diuretic and a calcium channel blocker is not particularly effective at controlling BP. In addition, increasing the dose of the calcium channel blocker may make the patient's lower limb oedema worse. Increasing the diuretic would then not be effective at reducing his oedema and may lead to deteriorating renal function. Stopping the amlodipine might lead to an improvement of the lower limb oedema The patient's renal function is not sufficiently impaired to contraindicate the use of ACE-I or A II RA. The change to an A II RA makes the patient's treatment more consistent with the British Hypertension Society guidelines, whereby patients over 55 are started on a CCB or a diuretic as first line medication (**55**). If this is not sufficient to control the patient's BP, an ACE-I /A II RA should be added. While a 24 hour BP could be useful at this stage, it should be performed if the BP is still not controlled after the patient's treatment has been optimized.

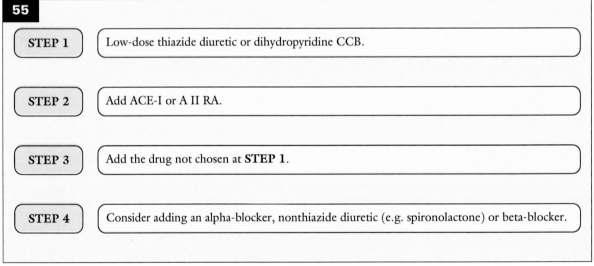

55

STEP 1	Low-dose thiazide diuretic or dihydropyridine CCB.
STEP 2	Add ACE-I or A II RA.
STEP 3	Add the drug not chosen at **STEP 1**.
STEP 4	Consider adding an alpha-blocker, nonthiazide diuretic (e.g. spironolactone) or beta-blocker.

55 Stepwise approach to drug treatment of hypertension in older people.

Patient 56

A 73-year-old man was admitted urgently with a stroke affecting the right side of his body. He was unable to speak and, the day after admission, he was unable to swallow. Hydration was maintained for the next 10 days with intravenous fluids while nasogastric feeding was attempted. However, he was unable to tolerate a nasogastric tube and pulled it out on two occasions when successful placement had been achieved; he appeared to be indicating that it was uncomfortable. On day 12 it was thought that his swallowing reflexes were improving, but attempts to provide nutrition over the next 11 days were not successful, culminating in an aspiration pneumonia. A decision was made to offer the patient a PEG which he accepted (he was able to understand speech and gave his assent to the treatment), though the placement of the PEG was delayed another 6 days while his chest cleared. Feeding through the PEG started on day 26 of the admission. Investigations performed on the day his PEG feeding started are shown.

A chest radiograph showed that the right lower lobe pneumonia was resolving and an ECG was normal. On day 29 of his admission he became dyspnoeic and drowsy. There appeared to be some generalized muscle tenderness and it was noted that he had oedema around his sacrum, ankles and, to some extent, hands. He was in atrial fibrillation with a ventricular rate of 90 bpm and a further chest radiograph showed evidence of early pulmonary oedema. His body temperature was normal and his oxygen saturation on air was 97%.

Investigations (normal range)

Haemoglobin 12.9 g/dL (13–18)
MCV 88 fL (80–99)
Total white cell count 11.2 × 10^9/L (4–11)
Neutrophil count 8.4 × 10^9/L (1.5–7)
Serum urea 2.1 mmol/L (2.5–7.5)
Serum sodium 139 mmol/L (137–144)
Serum potassium 3.9 mmol/L (3.5–4.9)
Serum creatinine 88 mmol/L (60–110)
Serum albumin 33 g/L (37–49)
Serum total bilirubin 22 mmol/L (1–22)
Serum ALT 21 U/L (5–35)
Serum alkaline phosphatase 80 U/L (45–105)

---

1 The most likely reason for his deterioration is:
 A Fluid overload.
 B MI.
 C Pulmonary embolism.
 D Septicaemia.
 E Refeeding syndrome.

---

2 The most useful next investigation under these circumstances is:
 A Serum troponin T and cardiac enzymes.
 B Serum phosphate and magnesium.
 C Echocardiogram.
 D Plasma insulin assay.
 E Serum sodium and potassium.

---

3 How should his condition be managed?

Patient 56 Answers

> **1 E** Refeeding syndrome.

The patient's deterioration has occurred 3 days after starting refeeding through the PEG tube. The clinical picture and the timing make it very likely that the patient has refeeding syndrome. He should be further investigated and managed along those lines unless there is firm evidence of an alternative cause for his worsening clinical status. Fluid overload is unlikely since the patient is now receiving nutrition and fluids through the PEG and he has normal renal function. However, fluid retention is a feature of the refeeding syndrome for reasons that are not fully understood. Myocardial infarction is always a possibility in patients in whom there is deterioration in clinical status accompanied by breathlessness; the onset of new atrial fibrillation can also be due to myocardial infarction. However, that diagnosis is less likely than refeeding syndrome and can easily be ruled out with appropriate investigations. Pulmonary embolism is unlikely in this patient as he is receiving prophylactic clexane and there has been no fall in his oxygen saturation. Similarly, there is little to support the diagnosis of sepsis, though if refeeding syndrome is not confirmed, sepsis should be considered.

> **2 B** Serum phosphate and magnesium.

The suspected diagnosis of refeeding syndrome would best be confirmed by measuring the serum phosphate and magnesium levels. It is characteristic of the syndrome to see an abrupt fall in the serum phosphate, magnesium and, sometimes, potassium as an acute event in the first few days after substantial quantities of carbohydrate are reintroduced to the patient's diet. Confirming the diagnosis quickly will enable the appropriate management to be put in place and the measured levels can be a guide to replacement therapies. Troponin T and cardiac enzymes would be helpful if MI is still considered to be a possibility and echocardiography would help to rule out a primary cardiac problem. However, it must be remembered that myocardial contractility may be impaired in patients with electrolyte disturbances caused by the refeeding syndrome. The plasma insulin level is likely to be high in any patient given carbohydrates after a period of fasting so measuring it does not help to establish the diagnosis. The serum sodium usually remains in the normal range providing fluid replacement has been satisfactory, though there may be a fall in the potassium level as part of the refeeding syndrome. However, this would not be as powerful evidence of that condition as a simultaneous fall in the phosphate and magnesium levels.

3 After a prolonged period of fasting it is advisable to reintroduce feeding, particularly carbohydrates, slowly. Usually, approximately a quarter of the estimated daily requirements would be given in the first few days, gradually increasing the amount towards the target level. If the reintroduction of feeding is conducted in that way, with monitoring of the phosphate and magnesium levels, a patient is unlikely to develop severe complications. In difficult cases clinicians should collaborate with dieticians and/or nutritionists to manage such patients. In the patient described it would be necessary to reduce the rate of feeding and give phosphate, magnesium, and potassium supplements to bring those indices into the normal range as quickly as possible. Of course, significant co-pathologies such as associated heart failure or sepsis should be dealt with accordingly.

Tutorial

The refeeding syndrome characteristically occurs when significantly malnourished patients are given nutritional supplements with a high carbohydrate content. There is a hyperinsulinaemic response to the reintroduction of carbohydrates with the rapid uptake of glucose into cells alongside insulin-mediated uptake of potassium and magnesium. Extracellular phosphate is then subsequently taken up by cells as they incorporate phosphate into high energy storage compounds such as adenosine triphosphate. Consequently, the serum concentration of phosphate ions can fall dramatically. It is thought that the rapid flux of phosphate, magnesium, and potassium ions into cells is responsible for the majority of the features of the refeeding syndrome, such as cardiac dysfunction and cardiac arrhythmias. There is a tendency to retain water and develop oedema, though the mechanism of that is uncertain.

In extreme cases the rapid increase in basal metabolic rate, with accompanying increase in cardiac workload, can cause cardiac decompensation, particularly in patients with very prolonged periods of malnutrition or with underlying cardiac disease. In such patients the refeeding syndrome can present as acute heart failure.

Another important dimension to the syndrome is GI food intolerance. This is thought to be due to atrophic changes in the GI mucosa and reduced production of digestive enzymes during the starvation phase. With the reintroduction of feeding, for example through a PEG tube, malabsorption occurs with consequent diarrhoea and sometimes vomiting. Rarer consequences of severe refeeding syndrome include rhabdomyolysis, seizures, haematological disorders, and multi organ failure. These complications are thought to be primarily mediated by the rapid fall in serum phosphate concentration.

Patient 57

An 89-year-old woman was referred to clinic because of declining mobility, generalized aches, and a recent fall. Her GP had made a provisional diagnosis of polymyalgia rheumatica when she was found to have an ESR of 40 mm/h and gave her prednisolone, though there was no improvement in her symptoms so the treatment was stopped. She lived alone and had been virtually housebound for about 3 years since she fell and fractured her left femur. She had refused outside help and her shopping was done fortnightly by a neighbour. She had not renewed her prescriptions for at least 2 years so took no medications. Her previous medical history included no other major illnesses. On examination she was fully conscious with an AMTS of 8/10. Pulse was 82 bpm and regular, heart sounds normal with no signs of cardiac failure. Examination of the chest revealed slight chest wall tenderness bilaterally but no other abnormal signs. The abdomen was normal as was the CNS. On skeleto-muscular system examination she was found to have very poor antigravity power, and on formal testing her quadriceps femoris muscles were reduced in power to 4/5 on the MRC scale. There was also possibly slight proximal muscle weakness in the upper limbs. Her muscles were not tender. Joint examination showed mild osteoarthrotic changes and some mild tenderness around knees, wrists, and elbows.

Her chest radiograph was reported as normal. A radiograph of the hips and knees was reported as being generally osteopenic with a left hemiarthroplasty but no visible fractures. Routine urine testing was negative for glucose, protein, blood, and leukocytes.

Investigations (normal range)

Haemoglobin 11.8 g/d/L (11.5–16.5)
White cell count 4.9×10^9/L (4–11)
ESR 36 mm/h (<30)
Serum urea 9.1 mmol/L (2.5–7.5)
Serum creatinine 125 µmol/L (60–110)
Serum sodium 143 mmol/L (137–144)
Serum potassium 4.0 mmol/L (3.5–4.9)
Serum corrected calcium 1.8 mmol/L (2.2–2.6)
Serum phosphate 0.8 mmol/L (0.8–1.4)
Serum albumin 38 g/L (37–49)
Serum total bilirubin 9 µmol/L (1–22)
Serum ALT 29 U/L (5–35)
Serum alkaline phosphatase 232 U/L (45–105)
Serum CK 56 U/L (24–170)
Plasma free thyroxine 15 pmol/L (10–22)

---

1 The most likely diagnosis in this patient is:
   A Polymyalgia rheumatica.
   B Polymyositis.
   C Osteomalacia.
   D Multiple myeloma.
   E Hyperparathyroidism.

---

2 Describe how you would manage this patient.

---

3 The most important underlying factor predisposing the patient to her recent deterioration is:
   A Renal impairment.
   B Age.
   C Malabsorption.
   D Housebound state.
   E Poor diet.

---

4 In the context of your working diagnosis, explain why the patient's serum phosphate level was in the normal range on presentation.

---

5 Over what timescale would you expect the patient's blood tests to return to normal after adequate treatment?

Patient 57 Answers

---

1 C Osteomalacia.

The clinical picture is most suggestive of osteomalacia. This diagnosis is supported by the patient's elderly, frail, housebound state, proximal muscle weakness and muscle aching, periarticular tenderness, low corrected serum calcium, and high serum alkaline phosphatase levels. Polymyalgia rheumatica is unlikely since the ESR is not particularly high and there is already a history of failure to respond to corticosteroid treatment. In polymyositis the patient would be expected to have more tender muscles, a higher ESR, and a high CK level. Multiple myeloma has to be considered in such a presentation, though it would be unusual for it to present with a low corrected serum calcium and relatively low ESR. Also, muscle tenderness and proximal muscle weakness is not normally a feature of myeloma. Patients with hyperparathyroidism are usually hypercalcaemic.

2 With the information available it would be reasonable to make a working diagnosis of vitamin D deficiency. Further supportive evidence could be obtained by demonstrating a low serum 25 hydroxy vitamin D concentration and raised parathyroid hormone level. In a patient such as the one described, there would be no need to wait for the results of such tests before starting vitamin D and calcium replacement therapy. The absence of overt osteomalacic changes on the radiographs, such as greenstick fractures or Looser's zones (57) by no means rules out the diagnosis and should not be a reason for delaying treatment. Indeed, in elderly patients with vitamin D deficiency, the majority will not have the classic radiological changes of osteomalacia. There is no universally agreed treatment regimen for replacing vitamin D in patients such as the one in this case study. When the biochemical changes are clear, it is usual to give a starting dose of ergocalciferol 7.5 mg

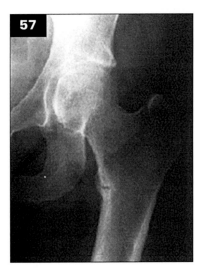

57 X-ray of the left hip showing a typical Looser's zone.

(300,000 U) as a single dose followed by calcium and vitamin D combined tablets containing 800 U of ergocalciferol daily. Some clinicians simply start a higher oral dose rather than give a depot. In patients with reasonably normal hepatic and renal function long-term prevention of overt vitamin D deficiency can be achieved in older patients with an 800 U/day supplement. Patients with malabsorption syndromes, chronic liver disease, and hypoparathyroidism often require much higher doses to achieve normocalcaemia. Once an elderly patient has presented with vitamin D deficiency, it is advisable to keep them on vitamin D and calcium supplements indefinitely.

---

3 D Housebound state.

In this patient the most important underlying factor predisposing her to the recent decline is her housebound state. Patients who have virtually no skin exposed to sunlight for many months at a time have no opportunity to generate vitamin D from precursors by the action of sunlight on skin. If they also have a diet marginal for vitamin D they gradually lapse into an overtly deficient state. Elderly housebound people in low sunlight areas are most prone but the risk also applies to housebound individuals in sunny climates. Patients with deeply pigmented skin are at additional risk. This patient's renal impairment was mild to moderate and would not be enough to prevent adequate renal conversion of vitamin D to the active form. Her age is in itself not a risk factor, though it does contribute indirectly because patients of great age are more likely to be housebound and have a diet that is marginal for a range of essential nutrients including vitamin D. There is no evidence in her clinical history or from her investigations to suggest she has a malabsorption state, though that should be considered in any patient with unexplained nutrient deficiencies. A poor diet is an important risk factor for osteomalacia and might apply in the case described, though there was not sufficient detail given about her diet to make that supposition.

4 The typical biochemical changes of osteomalacia include a low serum calcium and low serum phosphate level. This patient's serum phosphate was at the low end of the normal range and that is a common finding in older patients with osteomalacia and patients with osteomalacia related to renal impairment. This is thought to be due to reduced renal loss of phosphate in subjects with a lower GFR. Therefore, a serum phosphate in the normal range does not rule out osteomalacia.

5 With adequate vitamin D and calcium replacement, the patient's serum calcium and, if low, serum phosphate, would be expected to enter the normal range within 2–4

weeks. However, research has shown that the serum levels of those ions tends to continue to track towards the centre of the normal range for up to 1 year after starting treatment. The alkaline phosphatase concentration often initially rises after vitamin D supplements are given and then gradually falls over the course of about 12 months. The prolonged settling phase for these biochemical indices is thought to be related to the time required for bone to remodel fully after an adequate vitamin D status has been achieved.

Patient 58

A 94-year-old woman had been admitted to hospital four times in 5 months for the treatment of pneumonia. On each occasion she had received supportive treatments and antibiotics, and recovered sufficiently well to return to her sheltered housing. A diagnosis of Parkinson's disease had been made 2 years earlier, though she was taking no medication. There was no other significant medical history. On examination, she was slim and slightly lacked facial expression. Body temperature was 37.7°C. AMTS was 8/10, GCS, 15/15. Pulse was 94 bpm and regular, heart sounds normal and BP was 135/90 mmHg. The respiratory rate was 18 per minute and there were coarse crackles at the right lung base. No sputum was produced for inspection. Abdominal examination was normal and there were no focal neurological signs. Skeleto-muscular system was normal apart from a slight kyphosis and mild osteoarthrotic changes in her knees.

A chest radiograph showed patchy shadowing at the lung bases that was thought to be inflammatory (**58a**). Review of previous radiographs taken over the past 5 months showed patchy basal shadowing at both right and left lung bases at different times.

---

1 The most likely reason for this patient's clinical presentation is:
   A Underlying bronchogenic carcinoma.
   B Aspiration of oro-pharyngeal contents into airway.
   C Broncho-oesophageal fistula.
   D A failing immune system.
   E Basal bronchiectasis.

---

2 What might be the significance of the low haemoglobin and MCV in this context?

---

3 Which of the following investigations is most likely to yield diagnostic information?
   A CT scan of the thorax.
   B Bronchoscopy.
   C Gastroscopy.
   D Nonionic swallow contrast radiography.
   E Contrast bronchography.

---

4 What other baseline tests could be done to help to clarify the diagnosis?

Investigations (normal range)

Haemoglobin 10.1 g/dL (11.5–16.5)
MCV 76 fL (80–96)
Total white cell count 8.2 × 10⁹/L (4–11)
Neutrophil count 6.7 × 10⁹/L (1.5–7)
ESR 40 mm/h (<30)
Serum urea 7 mmol/L (2.5–7.5)
Serum sodium 140 mmol/L (137–144)
Serum potassium 4.2 mmol/L (3.5–4.9)
Serum total bilirubin 19 µmol/L (1–22)
Serum ALT 30 U/L (5–35)
Serum alkaline phosphatase 53 U/L (45–105)
Serum albumin 32 g/L (37–49)
Arterial blood gas analysis revealed:
pH 7.38 (7.36–7.44)
PO₂ (breathing air) 10.1 kPa (11.3–12.6)
PCO₂ 4.3 kPa (4.7–6)
Oxygen saturation 95%

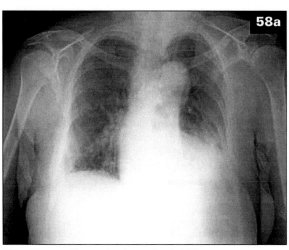

58a Chest radiograph taken after initial assessment.

Patient 58 Answers

---

1 B Aspiration of oro-pharyngeal contents into airway.

The most likely cause is aspiration of oro-pharyngeal secretions and food/drink into the airways. There is a number of features to suggest this as the most likely cause for this patient's clinical presentation. Firstly, she has had recurrent basal pneumonia; this is typical of recurrent aspiration, and there is some evidence that there is a predilection for aspiration into the right lower and middle lobes, though both lungs can be affected. The patient is elderly and there is an increasing prevalence of aspiration pneumonia due to an impairment of swallowing mechanisms with age. This is particularly likely to be seen in patients with cerebrovascular disease and extrapyramidal impairment. This patient had some evidence of Parkinson's disease, which is a risk factor for lung aspiration. An underlying bronchogenic carcinoma has always to be considered in patients with recurrent pneumonia. This is particularly important in patients where the pneumonia recurs in the same lobe, and is thought to be due to partial obstruction of the main airway to that lobe. There were no other features in this patient's presentation to support that suspicion. A broncho-oesophageal fistula would result, in most cases, in a more persistent pneumonia and the production of substantial amounts of sputum. Furthermore, such fistulae usually occur in the context of either bronchogenic or oesophageal malignancy. Recurrent pneumonia is a feature of patients with failing immunity, particularly those with underlying malignancies such as lymphoma and leukaemia and in acquired immunodeficiency states such as HIV/AIDS. In such patients the infecting organisms are often atypical or opportunistic and can be very difficult to treat. This patient recovered between episodes of basal pneumonia and had no other features to suggest a compromised immune state.

Bronchiectasis is an important cause of recurrent parenchymal lung inflammation, though in this patient the overall presentation was not typical of bronchiectasis as that condition would be expected to be accompanied by a history of daily production of a large volume of discoloured sputum over a long period of time, usually years.

2 Patients with an iron deficient state sometimes present with oesophageal motility disorders or the production of a mucosal web in the pharynx or oesophagus. The structural and functional changes that accompany that disorder can result in aspiration pneumonia. Therefore, it is important to check the iron status of any patient with unexplained dysphagia or oesophageal dysmotility, and the abnormalities are usually reversible if iron replacement therapy is given. Furthermore, an iron deficient state may be a mode of presentation for oesophageal malignancy or severe oesophageal ulceration, both of which can also be risk factors for aspiration into the airways through obstructive and reflux mechanisms respectively.

---

3 D Nonionic swallow contrast radiography.

A nonionic contrast swallow would provide the most certain diagnostic information in this patient. An example is seen in Figure **58b**. If significant amounts of the contrast medium enter the trachea and bronchi on swallowing, the case is proven. A CT scan of the thorax will confirm in more detail the inflammatory process at the bases and can detect obstructing mass lesions more accurately than plain chest radiography. However, it provides no information about the dynamic performance of the oesophagus and cannot demonstrate lack of functional integrity of the upper airway protective mechanism during swallowing. Bronchoscopy allows sampling of the inflamed area for bacteriological analysis and can detect intraluminal obstructing lesions in the airways. Failure of glottic closure during the procedure can also be helpful, and if aspiration is suspected, additional care is required not to introduce upper airway and pharyngeal material into the lower airways. Contrast bronchography is now rarely used, having been superseded by CT scanning for the diagnosis of bronchiectasis and it would not contribute any diagnostic information in a case such as the one described.

4 Assessing the safety of the swallowing mechanism at the bedside can be done with a high degree of reliability by observing the patient attempt to swallow water and observing the transfer of liquid to the back of the mouth and the fluency of the swallow. It is abnormal if coughing is induced or if coarse airway rattling is heard in the absence of cough. Additional information can be gleaned by monitoring oxygen saturation during the procedure. If

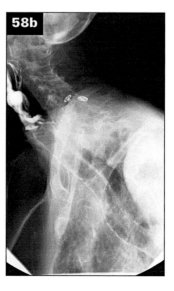

58b Nonionic contrast swallow showing aspiration of liquid into the upper airway.

oxygen saturation falls by 2% or more after swallowing between 10 and 20 ml of water, that is an indication of significant aspiration of water into the airways. The presence or absence of a gag reflex on touching the soft palate or uvula is not a reliable indicator of a safe swallowing mechanism. None of these bedside indications is as accurate as a nonionic contrast swallow with fluoroscopic screening.

Tutorial (Patient 58)

Most clinicians are familiar with overt aspiration of large amounts of foreign material such as food, drink, or vomit into the lungs. This causes a dramatic and serious form of pneumonia. In this context, the causation is usually apparent and the diagnosis straightforward. People of all ages are susceptible to such aspiration if their level of consciousness is reduced (particularly at risk if they have a GCS score of 9 or less). Recurrent small volume aspiration of the type described in the patient above is less well understood and can be missed in clinical practice if swallowing is not observed or formally assessed. In old age, particularly in patients with cerebrovascular disease, stroke, extrapyramidal disorders, or neuromuscular disorders, such low-volume aspiration is not at all uncommon. As in the case described, the patient can have several episodes of pneumonia before the causation is firmly established. The risk of aspiration pneumonia can be reduced by ensuring optimal control of conditions such as Parkinson's disease, advising the patient to sit in the upright position before attempting to swallow, and by thickening fluids to generate a quasi bolus response in some patients. The advice of a speech and language therapist is extremely valuable, particularly when there is some uncertainty about the condition in an individual patient and to obtain advice on management.

Patient 59

A 79-year-old man was referred to the Outpatient Clinic because of increasingly frequent falls and failing memory. His wife reported that he started having falls more than 2 years earlier, apparently due to a loss of balance and not being able to correct his balance in time. About 1 year later she first noticed his forgetfulness, and that symptom had become progressively worse. More recently, he had experienced occasional 'visions' of animals and small children. Sometimes he would lapse into an almost unrousable sleep for several hours in the afternoon. His only medication was amlodipine 5 mg daily for hypertension, which he had been taking for 9 years. On examination he looked well sitting in a chair. His AMTS was 6/10 and MMSE score 20/30. Pulse was 76 bpm and regular. Heart sounds were normal, BP 155/85 mmHg. Examination of the chest, abdomen, and skeleto-muscular system was normal for a man of his age. Nervous system examination showed some lack of facial expression and a reduced rate of blinking. The tone was slightly high in all limbs, though there was no asymmetry of tone. No tremor was observed and no cogwheel rigidity was elicited. His tendon reflexes were rather brisk but symmetrical and plantar reflexes were flexor. Sensory examination was normal. His gait was abnormal; he tended to take short steps and briefly festinated on turning. It was noted that he had an abnormal degree of body sway in the static and dynamic state and there was inadequate correction of his posture on the pull-back test of balance. His eye movements were normal.

Routine tests performed by his GP had shown that his full blood count, renal function, electrolytes, screening liver function and thyroid function tests were all normal as were an ECG and chest radiograph. A routine urine test in the clinic was also negative.

1 The diagnosis that best fits the description of this patient is:
A Alzheimer's disease.
B Parkinson's disease.
C Dementia with Lewy bodies.
D Multi infarct dementia.
E NPH.

2 If the visual hallucinations in this man were to become distressing, an appropriate drug regimen would be:
A Paroxetine.   D Quetiapine.
B Diazepam.   E L-dopa.
C Haloperidol.

3 Describe how you would manage his tendency to fall.

4 What problems might this patient face in the future?

Patient 59

Patient 59 Answers

> **1 C** Dementia with Lewy bodies.

The patient described shows many of the features suggestive of dementia with Lewy bodies. Of course, there is a substantial overlap between dementia with Lewy bodies, Alzheimer's disease, and Parkinson's disease. However, the initial presentation with postural instability, visual hallucinations, episodes of prolonged somnolence, and minimal (at this stage) extrapyramidal features, support the contention that this patient has dementia with Lewy bodies. Patients with Alzheimer's disease tend to present with the cognitive and behavioural problems dominating, and in idiopathic Parkinson's disease the extrapyramidal features usually appear first. Patients with multi infarct dementia vary in their presentation, according to the areas of damage, though visual hallucinations and excessive somnolence would be unusual in the early stages. The patient does not have the features of NPH, which, classically, presents with a shorter history, cognitive deficit, wide-based gait, and urinary incontinence. However, it remains on the list of differential diagnoses and would be one of the reasons for conducting a CT head scan in such a patient.

> **2 D** Quetiapine.

The visual hallucinations in Lewy body disease and in related disorders such as Alzheimer's disease and Parkinson's disease are sometimes brief and nonthreatening and require no medication. Indeed, patients sometimes retain insight into the fact that the visions are not real and can learn to disregard them. However, a proportion of patients will develop troublesome, persistent, and distressing visual hallucinations and can also develop other psychotic features such as delusions and auditory hallucinations. In Lewy body dementia the evidence is that such patients do best with an atypical antipsychotic drug such as quetiapine, starting at the lowest dose available and increasing as required. Although an atypical antipsychotic might potentiate the extrapyramidal features of Lewy body dementia, this is a relatively minor effect. Furthermore, the patient's main physical problem is the falls due to poor balance, rather than severe bradykinesia or tremor. There is no indication for a selective serotonin reuptake inhibitor such as paroxetine. Benzodiazepine tranquillizers such as diazepam would have an anxiolytic effect but would not suppress the hallucinations. Furthermore, they are likely to make the postural instability worse. Older antipsychotics such as haloperidol are more likely than the newer agents to exacerbate the extrapyramidal effects, and they are also more likely to cause other unwanted effects such as postural hypotension. There is no indication for L-dopa in the patient described at the moment, though some patients with Lewy body dementia in whom there are more pronounced Parkinsonian features can gain some benefit from L-dopa and dopamine agonist medications.

3 As described, the patient's tendency to fall is due to poor postural stability. The natural history of this would be to worsen gradually. Medications that might worsen the postural instability should be avoided whenever possible. If the patient's cognitive state allows it, he (and his carers) should be given advice on walking aids to improve postural stability. In the patient described, a wheeled Zimmer frame or delta rollator frame with brakes would probably be satisfactory. There should also be advice on how to avoid injury, largely through modification of his living environment. His carers should be given advice on how to assist him from the floor in the event of a fall and how to seek help under those circumstances.

4 The natural history of dementia with Lewy bodies is for the cognitive deficit, postural instability, Parkinsonian and psychotic features all to worsen. The patient and his carers need to be informed about this probable course of events and be given advice on how help can be provided to support independent living for as long as possible. If the patient has testamentary capacity, he or she should be advised that it would be sensible to make a will and, if desired, appoint an attorney in anticipation of loss of capacity in the future.

Patient 60

A 78-year-old woman became confused and agitated one evening and was brought to hospital by her nephew. She was unable to give a coherent history. The nephew reported that his aunt had not been really well for several weeks and had been complaining of a poor appetite, weight loss of at least 6 kg, increasing breathlessness, and a lump on her head that had bled on occasions. She had refused to see her general practitioner. She had a history of a cholecystectomy many years earlier and thyrotoxicosis, for which she had received radioactive iodine, 3 years ago. Her only medication was thyroxine 100 µg daily. On examination she was afebrile and it was not possible to perform the AMTS because she was unable to concentrate sufficiently. There was a painless ulcerated nodule on her scalp (60a) and several similar lesions on her chest, shoulder (60b), and upper arm. Some of these skin lesions had a slightly depressed centre giving them a dimpled appearance. Her pulse was 90 bpm and regular, heart sounds normal. BP was 160/90 mmHg. Respiratory rate was 18 per minute and there was dullness to percussion and reduced air entry at the left lung base. Her oxygen saturation was 96% on air. Abdominal examination was normal and there were no obvious focal CNS signs. Examination of the breasts revealed no definite masses.

An ECG was reported as normal and a chest radiograph showed a moderate-sized left pleural effusion.

Investigations (normal range)

Haemoglobin 8.9 g/dL (11.5–16.5)
MCV 90 fL (80–96)
Total white cell count 7.2 × 10^9/L (4–11)
ESR 54 mm/hr (<20)
Serum urea 7.8 mmol/L (2.5–7.5)
Serum creatinine 90 mmol/L (60–110)
Serum sodium 141 mmol/L (137–144)
Serum potassium 4.3 mmol/L (3.5–4.9)
Serum chloride 106 mmol/L (95–107)
Serum corrected calcium 3.6 mmol/L (2.2–2.6)
Serum phosphate 1.1 mmol/L (0.8–1.4)
Serum albumin 32 g/L (37–49)
Serum total bilirubin 4 mmol/L (1–22)
Serum ALT 29U/L (5–35)
Serum alkaline phosphatase 184 U/L (45–105)
Random plasma glucose 4.2 mmol/L
Serum urate 0.43 mmol/L (0.19–0.36)
Plasma free thyroxine 14 pmol/L (10–22)

---

1 Judging from their appearance and the clinical context, the most likely cause of the skin lesions is:
   A Tophaceous gout.
   B Neurofibromatosis.
   C Calcified parasites.
   D Sarcoma.
   E Metastases.

2 The acute confusion is most likely to be due to:
   A Hyperuricaemia.
   B Anaemia.
   C Hypercalcaemia.
   D Dehydration.
   E Sepsis.

3 In this patient, what else might be contributing to the acute confusional state?

4 Describe how you would proceed with investigation of the patient to establish the diagnosis.

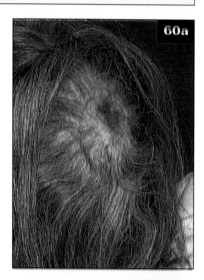

60a Painless ulcerated lesion on the scalp.

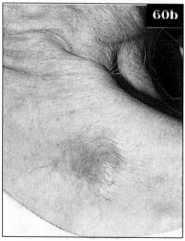

60b Lesion present on the shoulder.

Patient 60 Answers

---

1 E Metastases.

The skin lesions are about 2 cm in diameter and some have a dimpled centre, suggesting central necrosis. They are painless and are distributed apparently randomly. Furthermore, the patient has constitutional symptoms such as a poor appetite and weight loss. This suggests that metastatic spread to the skin from a primary tumour is the most likely reason for the nodules. Central ulceration is also suggestive of the diagnosis, particularly if the patient has been tempted to pick at the lesion, such as has happened with the scalp lesion in the patient described.

Tophaceous gout does not have this appearance. It typically occurs in the subcutaneous tissues adjacent to joints, particularly in the hands and feet, in the fleshy parts of the fingers and toes and in the pinnae of the ears. Neurofibromatosis is an inherited disorder and, by late adult life, the patient would have had skin neurofibromata for many years, along with other features such as café au lait spots. Furthermore, the lesions do not have the appearance of skin neurofibromata. Calcified parasites can cause subcutaneous nodules, particularly if they calcify, though this is a very slow process and would not be expected to be associated with constitutional symptoms. Furthermore, subcutaneous sequestration of parasites is uncommon in temperate climates. A sarcoma has to be considered with any unexplained nodular skin lesion. However, this patient's lesions do not have the appearance of Kaposi's sarcoma and most other sarcomata associated with skin would be solitary.

---

2 C Hypercalcaemia.

In this patient the most likely reason for the onset of the confusional state is hypercalcaemia. Older patients with corrected serum calcium levels above 3 mmol/L will often have some degree of confusion. As a broad rule of thumb, if the corrected serum calcium is less than 3 mmol/L, confusion is much less likely to occur and if it is above 4 mmol/L in an older person, a confusional state is usual. Hyperuricaemia does not cause a confusional state. This patient is not sufficiently anaemic to compromise cerebral oxygenation, though anaemia may be a contributing factor. There is no evidence that she is dehydrated or septic.

3 In the patient described the possibility of metastatic brain disease has to be considered in the differential diagnosis of the confusional state. Some patients with metastatic disease present with the gradual onset of focal neurological loss, though it is not uncommon for such patients to present with an acute confusional state. Although no evidence of sepsis has been presented in the information above, it would be good practice to keep the possibility of infection in mind, particularly if the confusional state does not resolve with correction of the serum calcium level. Some patients with significant degrees of sepsis do not mount a febrile or leukocytic response, and there is some evidence that this is particularly likely in older people with underlying malignant disease.

4 It is necessary to establish a tissue diagnosis in order to plan the management of this patient. As several skin lesions are easily accessible, needle biopsy or excision biopsy would be the most straightforward method of obtaining a histological diagnosis. In the patient above, the diagnosis proved to be metastatic carcinoma of the breast and there was significant benefit from hormonal therapy. The lack of an apparent primary tumour on bedside examination of the breasts does not deflect from the diagnosis. Sometimes the primary is small, as was the case in this patient, or may have been removed surgically many years before. If the patient's confusional state does not improve with correction of the hypercalcaemia (in this case with fluids and pamidronate), it would be sensible to obtain a CT head scan to look for brain metastases. A case can be made for performing further tests to diagnose the cause of the pleural effusion. Thoracocentesis sometimes yields useful cytology. Intrathoracic metastases can be detected by CT scanning.

Patient 61

An 83-year-old woman was referred for urgent inpatient assessment because she had fallen twice in 24 hours and had caused a fire in her kitchen. She was a widow who had lived alone for many years, managing independently and doing her own shopping until 2 weeks before presentation. Neighbours had noticed that she had been talking 'rubbish' and seemed bewildered for about 2 weeks, and had therefore contacted the patient's general practitioner. The patient had suffered in a concentration camp in World War II, during which time she worked for several months on a boiler construction project. She had a 45 pack-year smoking history but gave up 6 years ago. There was also a record of a right mastectomy having been performed 22 years early for carcinoma of the breast,

though there had never been any evidence of metastatic disease. Her only medications were salbutamol and ipratropium metered-dose inhalers for use as required.

On examination she was disorientated in time and place. Her AMTS was 2/10. She was afebrile with no lymphadenopathy. Pulse was 86 bpm and regular, BP 115/70 mmHg, auscultation of the heart revealed a quiet mitral pansystolic murmur, and her JVP was not raised. Her respiratory rate was 16 per minute and auscultation of the chest revealed expiratory rhonchi and a few coarse basal lung crackles symmetrically. Examination of the abdomen and skeleto-muscular system was normal. There were no obvious focal CNS signs, though that aspect of the examination was limited by her confused state. A routine specimen of urine tested positive for blood and leukocytes.

An ECG showed nonspecific T wave changes only and her chest radiograph is shown (61).

Investigations (normal range)

Haemoglobin 11.5 g/dL (11.5–16.5)
MCV 88 fL (80–96)
Total white cell count 6.3×10^9/L (4–11)
ESR 63 mm/hr (<30)
Serum urea 3.6 mmol/L (2.5–7.5)
Serum sodium 112 mmol/L (137–144)
Serum potassium 3.6 mmol/L (3.5–4.9)
Serum chloride 90mmol/L (95–107)
Serum corrected calcium 2.4 mmol/L (2.2–2.6)
Serum albumin 38 g/L (37–49)
Serum total bilirubin 14 µmol/L (1–22)
Serum ALT 30 U/L (5–35)
Serum alkaline phosphatase 59 U/L (45–105)
Plasma free thyroxine 17 pmol/L (10–22)
Fasting plasma glucose 10.4 mmol/L (3–6)
Arterial PO_2 breathing air 10.9 kPa (11.3–12.6)
Arterial PCO_2 5.1 kPa (4.7–6.0)
pH 7.39 (7.36–7.44)

---

61 Chest radiograph taken at initial assessment.

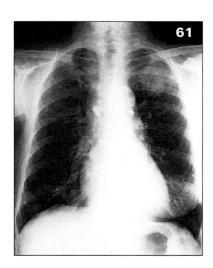

---

1 The most likely cause of her confusional state is:
   A Hyponatremia.
   B Cerebral metastases.
   C UTI.
   D Diabetic precoma.
   E Pneumonia.

---

2 The lesion on the chest radiograph is most likely to be:
   A An asbestos plaque.
   B Bronchogenic carcinoma.
   C Metastatic breast cancer.
   D Lung abscess.
   E TB.

---

3 The initial management of her electrolyte disturbance should be:
   A Intravenous hypertonic saline.
   B Demeclocyclin.
   C Fluid restriction.
   D Oral balanced salt solution.
   E Oral frusemide.

---

4 The mechanism of the electrolyte disturbance can best be ascertained for clinical purposes by:
   A Measuring urinary chloride concentration.
   B Urine and plasma osmolality.
   C Calculating the anion gap.
   D Assaying plasma ADH.
   E Conducting a demeclocyclin challenge test.

Patient 61 Answers

1 A Hyponatremia.

In this clinical context the most likely reason for the patient's presentation is hyponatremia. Most elderly patients with a serum sodium as low as 112 mmol/L have some degree of confusion. If the serum sodium level has fallen relatively quickly, a confusional state is almost inevitable. Cerebral metastases must be considered in this patient because of the history of breast cancer and the abnormal appearance of the chest radiograph. However, there were no other clinical features to support that diagnosis in this case. There is no good evidence for UTI in this patient. The presence of blood and leukocytes on a routine specimen of urine is weak evidence for a significant lower UTI. Furthermore, the patient was neither febrile nor had a leukocytosis and did not complain of any dysuric symptoms. Although the patient had a high fasting blood sugar and was likely to have a degree of glucose intolerance, there was no other evidence of diabetic precoma and the pH was in the normal range. A diagnosis of pneumonia would be difficult to sustain in this patient since there were no appropriate symptoms and no epiphenomena of sepsis on investigation. In addition, the chest radiograph appearance was not that of pneumonia.

2 B Bronchogenic carcinoma.

The appearance of the patient's chest radiograph is strongly supportive of a diagnosis of bronchogenic carcinoma. The image shows a rounded abnormality in the left apical zone, possibly with some central necrosis. Furthermore, the patient has other risk factors including a history of smoking, her age, and the possibility that she may have been exposed to asbestos during boiler construction work in her youth. The appearances are not those of an asbestos plaque. Metastatic disease from the breast cancer is a possibility, though remote, because of the lack of any other evidence of late relapse of the breast cancer. A lung abscess is a possibility, though the lesion looks rather too radio-dense for that diagnosis. Patients with lung abscesses almost always have a fever and leukocytosis and a productive cough. Apical lung shadowing always raises the possibility of tuberculosis, though the appearance in this patient is not that of a typical tuberculous apical lung lesion.

3 C Fluid restriction.

The initial management should be aimed at correcting the hyponatremia. In the first instance this would be best started by restricting the patient's 24 hour fluid intake to 1.2 L, reducing to 1 L or even lower if the response is inadequate. Ideally, the patient's serum sodium would rise gradually by 2–3 mmol/day; a faster rise can cause further decompensation of the patient's mental state. As the serum sodium rises, the patient's sensorium would be expected to clear, though there is sometimes a lag between reaching the normonatraemic range and a return to normal cognition.

The patient is most likely to have SIADH due to ectopic production from the lung cancer. This results in retention of water at renal level with a dilutional hyponatraemia. Giving intravenous hypertonic saline would have no effect and can be dangerous in that it can precipitate volume overload. Demeclocyclin is a useful drug in this context. It is a tetracycline that is thought to block the action of ADH on renal tubules. In patients who do not respond to fluid restriction, it is a useful means of bringing the serum sodium into the normal range. Most patients, particularly those with reversible causes of SIADH, do not require it, though some patients with untreatable underlying causes (as might be the case in the patient described) can require demeclocyclin for long-term management. However, it would not be the first line of treatment. Balanced salt solutions would have no effect and, if anything, would add to the water load. Diuretic treatment would result in some loss of salt and water but would not be expected to correct the serum sodium concentration.

4 B Urine and plasma osmolality.

In everyday clinical practice, the presence of SIADH is best demonstrated by measuring the urine and plasma osmolality. If the plasma osmolality is below the normal range while the urine osmolality is inappropriately high, the diagnosis is supported. Some older people who are unable to concentrate their urine because of impaired renal function (renal medullary dysfunction), sometimes fall slightly short of the strict criteria and that must be borne in mind when interpreting the results. Urinary chloride measurement is rarely performed in modern practice. It would not be of help in managing this patient. In desalinated patients with, for example, severe GI fluid loss or heat stroke, the urinary chlorides tend to be absent and their reappearance in urine is an early indication of adequate repletion with sodium chloride.

Little would be gained by calculating the anion gap in the patient described as there is no evidence of a significant acid-based disorder. Demonstrating an inappropriately high plasma ADH in the face of a low serum osmolality would be strong evidence to support the diagnosis of SIADH. However, the assay is time-consuming and is therefore rarely of use in clinical practice. There is no formal protocol for a demeclocycline challenge test. However, some clinicians give demeclocycline and track the response as a means of supporting the diagnosis of SIADH in patients where there is still some diagnostic uncertainty.

Patient 62

A 74-year-old man was referred because of inability to sleep. This had led to a profound feeling of daytime tiredness and a persistent depressed affect. On direct questioning he revealed that he had constant itching in all parts of his body but particularly his shoulders, trunk, and the upper part of his legs. This had caused him some embarrassment and he had not mentioned it to his GP. At first he thought he had scabies but a trial of two different treatments purchased from his local pharmacist had led to no improvement. He also said that a similar rash had occurred about 10 years earlier, which lasted 3–4 weeks and cleared spontaneously. He was otherwise well. There was a history of asthma, though that had rarely been a problem in recent years, and he took no medication. On examination he was afebrile and looked well. There were no abnormal physical signs except the rash shown in Figure **62**. This was visible on his abdomen and back, shoulders, upper arms, and around his buttocks and the top of his thighs. Upper body flexures such as the axillae and groins were not affected and there was no sign of the rash on his hands, feet, or head.

Investigations performed recently by his GP were normal including a full blood count, renal function tests, electrolytes, basic liver function tests, thyroid hormone level, and chest radiograph.

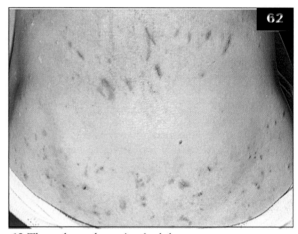

62 The rash on the patient's abdomen.

1 In this clinical context the rash (**62**) was most likely to be due to:
A Scabies.
B Body lice.
C Psoriasis.
D Eczema.
E Fungal infection.

2 How should this patient be treated initially?

3 What predisposes older patients to this condition?

Patient 62 Answers

---

1 D Eczema.

It is most likely that this rash is due to eczema. The distribution on shoulders, trunk, and around the hips and thighs suggests that it might be due to a contact dermatitis caused by, for example, biological washing powder. The absence of the rash from areas not in contact with clothes suggests that that might be the case. Scabies remains a possibility with a rash of this appearance, though the failure to respond to two different scabies treatments and the lack of other features of scabies such as interdigital tracks make that diagnosis less likely. The appearance and time course of the condition does not suggest psoriasis. Body lice and fungal infections would normally favour enclosed body folds such as the axillae, groins and, in women and obese men, the area beneath the breasts.

2 If a provisional diagnosis of probable eczema is made, there should be an enquiry as to whether any new potential allergens have been introduced into the patient's environment. In the patient described in this example, it was found that a new washing powder was being employed for his washing and his symptoms resolved progressively after that source of irritation was removed. If no obvious allergen can be identified, it is often possible to manage the patient with plain emollients, a reduction in the use of soap when bathing (thereby allowing the skin to be less depleted of oils), and the prescription of an antipruritic agent, particularly at night. Antihistamines are very effective for such patients. A nonsedating antihistamine can be used by day and a sedating formulation such as chlorpheniramine can be used at night to promote sleep. Some patients require low-dose topical corticosteroid treatments and a small proportion will require oral systemic steroids to bring the condition under control. If the patient has persisting or difficult symptoms, and particularly if there is still doubt about the diagnosis, a specialist opinion should be sought from a dermatologist.

3 Older patients may be predisposed to eczema by a number of factors. Some of these are the same for patients of all ages, such as an atopic tendency. However, ageing skin is drier and more prone to cracking. This can lead to direct chemical irritation of the skin structures and allows entry of allergens. Older patients' skin is also more likely to be dried out by the use of soaps, detergents, and solvents.

Tutorial

In eczema the main problems occur in the epidermis where skin cells become less tightly bound. This allows ingress of irritant chemicals that exacerbate the condition further. There is almost always severe itching under these circumstances causing the patient to rub or scratch the skin, leading to further mechanical damage. In fact, scratch marks can be easily seen in Figure **62**. Thus, an itch–scratch cycle sets in which potentiates the skin lesion and prevents healing. Patients who are prone to eczema often have an atopic history and associated atopic clinical syndromes such as asthma, allergic rhinitis, or a history of classical childhood flexural eczema. Patients with eczema exhibit exaggerated (mainly Type I) immune responses to allergens in the skin with release of inflammatory mediators including histamine. It is thought that damage to the mechanical integrity of skin leads to a potential for hypersensitivity to bacterial allergens that can then potentiate a chronic eczematous state.

Patient 63

A 78-year-old woman was referred with acute confusion and incontinence of urine. The symptoms had been present for about 3 days. Before that, she lived alone independently in a flat but was unable to walk and used a wheelchair. No other information was available to the admitting team. Her previous medical history was unknown but she brought the following medications: prednisolone 10 mg daily, auranofin 6 mg daily, paracetamol 1 g three times daily.

On examination she had a tympanic membrane temperature of 37.9°C. There was no lymphadenopathy and she was not pale. She was disorientated in time and place and her AMTS was 3/10. Her pulse was 94 bpm and regular, heart sounds normal, BP 130/75 mmHg, JVP normal, respiratory rate 22 per minute, and coarse crackles could be heard throughout both lungs. Examination of the abdomen was normal. CNS examination was difficult because of her confusion but no obvious focal or lateralizing signs were found. Skeleto-muscular examination showed multiple small joint deformities of the hands and feet (**63a**) and severe valgus deformities of both knees. Her hips were both stiff and painful and she was not able to extend them easily beyond the 90° position. None of the joints appeared to be acutely inflamed. Shortly after her physical examination was complete, she coughed and expectorated a large volume of greenish-brown sputum.

An ECG showed no significant abnormalities. Her chest radiograph is shown (**63b**).

Investigations (normal range)

Haemoglobin 9.3 g/dL (11.5–16.5)
Total white cell count 2.8 × 10⁹/L (4–11)
Neutrophil count 1.4 × 10⁹/L (1.5–7)
Platelet count 75 × 10⁹/L (150–400)
ESR 90 mm/h (<30)
Serum urea 13.2 mmol/L (2.5–7.5)
Serum creatinine 121 µmol/L (60–110)
Serum sodium 138 mmol/L (137–144)
Serum potassium 4.7 mmol/L (3.5–4.9)
Serum corrected calcium 2.5 mmol/L (2.2–2.6)
Serum albumin 31g/L (37–49)
Serum total bilirubin 15 µmol/L (1–22)
Serum ALT 31 U/L (5–35)
Serum alkaline phosphatase 48 U/L (45–105)
Plasma free thyroxine 13 pmol/L (10–22)
Arterial PO_2 (breathing air) 8.4 kPa (11.3–12.6)
Arterial PCO_2 4.9 kPa (4.7–6)
Arterial pH 7.41 (7.36–7.44)
Random plasma glucose 4.2 mmol/L

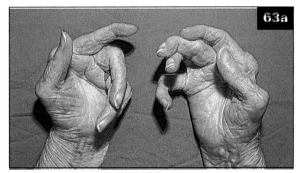

63a The patient's hands.

1 Describe the hand abnormalities in Figure **63a**. What is the most likely cause?

2 What does the chest radiograph (**63b**) show? How might the lesions be related to the joint disease?

3 Why is the patient incontinent?

4 Which of the following is the most appropriate intervention at this stage:
   A Platelet transfusion.
   B Infliximab.
   C Fresh frozen plasma.
   D Parenteral corticosteroids.
   E Antibiotics.

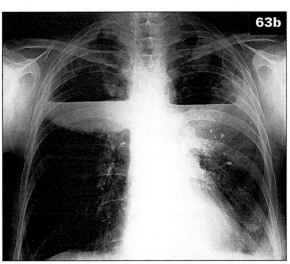

63b Chest radiograph of patient presenting with confusion, cough, and sputum.

Patient 63 Answers

1 The patient's hands show clear ulnar deviation at the MTP joints, wasting of the muscles of the hands, and spindling of the fingers. This appearance is virtually diagnostic of RA. Other typical signs in the hands would be swan neck and boutonnière deformities in the fingers, subluxation of the wrist joint, and weakness. If the joints are actively inflamed, there will be swelling, redness, and tenderness over the joints and there may also be tenosinovitis, particularly involving the tendons around the wrists.

2 The chest radiograph shows bilateral large apical cavities with inflammatory changes in the cavity walls and distinct fluid levels. These appearances are characteristic of bilateral apical lung abscesses. RA is associated with a number of pulmonary lesions, the commonest of which is pleural effusion from an associated serositis, diffuse fibrosing alveolitis, though this is relatively uncommon, rheumatoid lung nodules and, rarely, obliterative bronchiolitis. Patients with industrial dust diseases can develop a more florid nodular pulmonary fibrosis known as Kaplan's syndrome. However, there is no direct association between RA and apical lung abscesses. Nevertheless, there is extensive evidence that this patient could have a deficient immune system. The rheumatoid disease itself can cause some suppression of immunity but it is more likely that the combined treatment with prednisolone and gold are causing immunosuppression in this patient. It is likely that the low white cell count, neutropenia, and thrombocytopenia are due to the gold therapy; a neutropenia of this level could be contributing to insufficient defence against bacterial infection. The gold therapy could also be suppressing cell-mediated immunity through reduced macrophage function. The nonspecific presentation with confusion and incontinence in this patient is not unusual in older patients with serious pulmonary infection. Furthermore, in the immunosuppressed state, the patient often has more advanced disease at the time of presentation because symptoms are less florid.

3 It is difficult to say for certain which factor is predominantly responsible for this patient's incontinence. This is very typical of the acute onset of incontinence in a frail older person. The patient is sufficiently hypoxic for cerebral hypoxia to be contributing to the confusional state, with incontinence of urine as a secondary phenomenon. The patient's immobility also makes it very difficult for her to use toilet facilities. Furthermore, the patient's toxic state as a result of an acute febrile infectious illness could also be contributing to the confusion and incontinence synergistically with the hypoxia.

63c Improvement of the lung abscesses after 2 weeks of antibiotic treatment.

---

4 E Antibiotics.

As discussed in the last question, the root cause of the patient's presenting problems is infection. Therefore, in addition to basic supportive care, the most appropriate intervention is to give antibiotics for the lung abscesses. It is necessary to cover common respiratory bacterial pathogens and anaerobic infection with a combination such as amoxicillin and metronidazole, though local bacteriological advice should be sought under these circumstances. Most lung abscesses will clear with antibiotic therapy, usually leaving a parenchymal lung scar. Figure **63c** shows partial resolution after 2 weeks of treatment. There is no indication to give a platelet transfusion since the platelet count in this patient is only moderately reduced and there are no clinical features of thrombocytopenia. Similarly, fresh frozen plasma is not indicated as it would not contribute significantly to the antibacterial therapy and the patient, despite a slightly low albumin, has no features of hypoproteinemia. Infliximab has been used in some circumstances with overwhelming or difficult infection for its antitumour necrosis factor effect. However, there is no indication to give it before or alongside antibiotics in this patient and there will be no need to use it for the rheumatoid disease in such a patient, as all the indications are that the RA itself is adequately controlled on current therapy. There is no indication to give parenteral corticosteroids since there is nothing to suggest that the patient has clinical features of corticosteroid lack and it would make no contribution to the control of the patient's underlying infection.

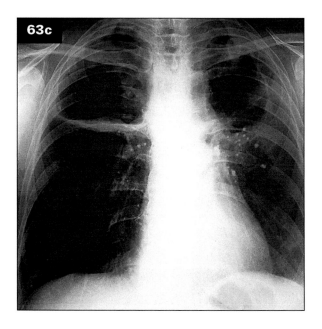

Tutorial (Patient 63)

Frail elderly patients taking immunosuppressive therapies for conditions such as RA not infrequently fall out of follow-up as a result of the difficulties they experience attending clinics. Under those circumstances the patient can drift into a critically immunocompromised state and present with significant infections, such as in the patient described above, or with other side-effects of the same group of drugs, such as bone marrow suppression. The most important drugs in this context are methotrexate, azathioprine, cyclosporin, cylophosphamide, leflunomide, and the cytokine inhibitors such as infliximab. Corticosteroids should also be thought of in the same way. Close cooperation is required between secondary and primary care to ensure adequate monitoring of frail elderly patients taking such medications.

Patient 64

A 75-year-old woman presented with sudden onset of sharp central chest pain radiating to her back. She collapsed with a BP of 80/50 mmHg in the right arm and unrecordable BP in the left arm. A CT scan of her chest and abdomen is shown below (**64a, 64b**).

1 What is the diagnosis?
  A Acute massive pulmonary embolism.
  B Ruptured oesophagus.
  C Dissection of the aorta.
  D Massive MI.
  E Tension pneumothorax.

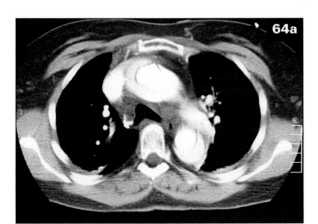

64a CT chest scan from patient presenting with chest pain.

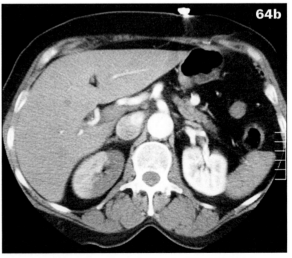

64b CT abdomen scan at the level of the kidneys.

Patient 64 Answer

1 **C** Dissection of the aorta.

The CT scan in Figure **64a** shows a massive dissection of the ascending aorta and arch. A flap is present in the aorta (arrows in Figure **64c**) generating a false lumen. In Figure **64b** one can see that the dissection extends down the descending aorta involving the right renal artery causing infarction of the right kidney (arrow in Figure **64d**). Unfortunately the patient died before any treatment could be given.

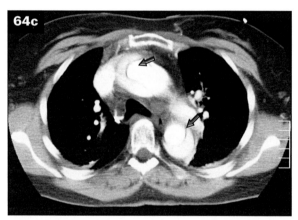

64c CT chest scan showing dissection of the ascending aorta and arch.

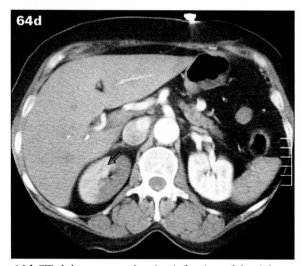

64d CT abdomen scan showing infarction of the right kidney.

Tutorial

Aortic dissection is a condition that involves bleeding into and along the wall of the aorta because of a tear or damage to the inner surface of the artery. This usually occurs in the thoracic portion of the aorta, but may also occur in the abdominal portion. Aortic dissection occurs in approximately 2 out of every 10,000 people. It can affect anyone, but is most often seen in men aged 40–70 (*Table 64*).

The risk of death is highest for aneurysms involving the ascending aorta. For that reason, most of those aneurysms receive urgent surgical attention. Dissections of the descending thoracic aorta can often be treated with BP control. The medical treatment includes aggressive control of BP and heart rate while the aorta heals. The risk of death with medical treatment of descending thoracic aortic dissection is about 10%. If surgery is required, the risk rises to about 30%.

Once the acute dissection has healed, adequate control of BP may eliminate the need for surgery. Lifelong monitoring of the aortic diameter is required, because a previously dissected descending thoracic aorta may enlarge and rupture.

The risk of undergoing surgery for an ascending aortic dissection is also significant. The risk is less for people who come to the operating room in good condition, and greatest for those who are in shock when they undergo surgery.

Table 64 *Risk factors for aortic dissection*
- Atherosclerosis
- Hypertension
- Trauma (especially blunt trauma such as hitting a steering wheel in a car accident)
- Infection, e.g. syphilitic aortitis
- Congenital weakness of the aortic wall
- Collagen disorders (Marfan's syndrome, Ehlers–Danlos syndrome)
- Relapsing polychondritis
- Pregnancy
- Valvular heart disease (particularly aortic regurgitation)
- Coarctation of the aorta

Patient 65

A 79-year-old woman came to hospital as an emergency, complaining of abdominal pain. This had been present on and off for about 4 days, becoming increasingly severe. She had taken codeine (prescribed for her husband) for the pain without much benefit. On the day before admission she had two falls and a 1-hour period of acute confusion. She remained able to drink and there had been no vomiting or diarrhoea. Her health was previously excellent and, until the onset of this illness, she had never been admitted to hospital. Her medical history consisted of minor illnesses only and she was taking no medication. On examination she was afebrile, pulse 88 bpm and regular, heart sounds normal, BP 135/85 mmHg, respiratory rate 12 per minute, and examination of the chest was normal. Abdominal examination revealed mild generalized tenderness throughout the abdomen with no guarding, no masses, and normal bowel sounds. A rash was noted across her buttocks (65). This was a nonblanching, slightly raised, nontender rash that the patient's husband reported had first been noticed about 2 days before admission. CNS examination was normal except for the slight confusion, and skeleto-muscular system examination revealed slightly swollen and tender knees but was otherwise normal.

Her chest radiograph was reported as normal. An ECG was also normal. A routine specimen of urine tested positive for protein and red blood cells but was otherwise normal.

A biopsy of the rash revealed leukocytoclastic infiltration of blood vessel walls.

Investigations (normal range)

Haemoglobin 12.4 g/dL (11.5–16.5)
White cell count 12.2 × 10^9/L (4–11)
Neutrophil count 7.9 × 10^9/L (1.5–7)
Eosinophil count 0.8 × 10^9/L (0.04–0.4)
Platelet count 320 × 10^9/L (150–400)
ESR 25 mm/h (<30)
Serum urea 7.9 mmol/L (2.5–7.5)
Serum creatinine 76 µmol/L (60–110)
Serum sodium 139 mmol/L (137–144)
Serum potassium 3.8 mmol/L (3.5–4.9)
Serum albumin 46 g/L (37–49)
Serum total bilirubin 14 µmol/L (1–22)
Serum ALT 31 U/L (5–35)
Serum alkaline phosphatase 60 U/L (45–105)
Fasting plasma glucose 4.1 mmol/L (3–6)
Plasma free thyroxine 14 pmol/L (10–22)

Investigations obtained later in the admission included:

Serum CRP 12 mg/L (<10)
ANCA negative
Antinuclear antibodies negative
Antigastric parietal cell antibody negative
Antimitochondrial antibody negative
Antismooth muscle antibody negative
Rheumatoid factor 16 kU/L (<30)

---

1 The most likely cause of the rash is:
   A Meningococcal septicaemia.
   B Henoch-Schönlein purpura.
   C Idiopathic thrombocytopenic purpura.
   D Bacterial endocarditis.
   E Systemic lupus erythematosus.

---

2 What is the most likely reason for her to present with falls and confusion?

---

3 How should the condition be managed?

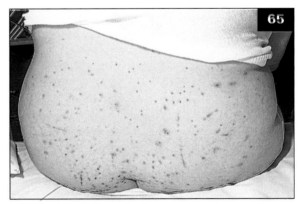

65 The rash on the patient's buttocks and upper thighs.

Patient 65 Answers

---

1 B Henoch-Schönlein purpura.

If this patient had presented at the age of 10 years there would have been little difficulty in making the diagnosis of Henoch-Schönlein purpura. That condition is usually seen in children and young adults, though older patients with an identical clinical syndrome have been described. This is one such patient. The diagnosis at the time of presentation was supported by the presence of the purpuric rash around the buttocks and the upper part of the legs, abdominal pain, and bilateral painful knees. (The triad of lower limb purpura, abdominal pain, and arthritis is the classical presentation in young patients.) There is no evidence to suggest that the patient had meningococcal septicaemia. In such a case the rash would not usually be localized and there would be more evidence of infection such as a more definite leukocytosis and fever. By definition, the patient did not have idiopathic thrombocytopenic purpura because the platelet count was normal. There were no features to support the diagnosis of bacterial endocarditis, in which a vasculitic rash is usually sparse and not localized, and though a vasculitic rash can be seen in systemic lupus, there was no other clinical or serological evidence to support that diagnosis. Later on in the admission, the finding of a negative autoimmune screen, normal erythrocyte sedimentation rate and marginal C-reactive protein, together with the leukocytoclastic vasculitic picture on biopsy provided further support for the diagnosis.

2 The patient was most likely to have developed a confusional state because she had self-medicated herself with codeine. This, plus her painful knees, would have contributed to her tendency to fall. She had been able to continue to take fluids during this illness so it was unlikely that she was significantly dehydrated. That interpretation was supported by the normal urea and electrolyte levels. Henoch-Schönlein purpura is not associated with cerebral vasculitis.

3 There is no specific treatment for Henoch-Schönlein purpura. Supportive measures are important as are analgesics for the abdominal pain. There is some evidence that patients with abdominal pain can be helped with systemic corticosteroid treatment and adults severely affected by the GI complications have been shown to benefit from treatment with Factor VIII concentrate. Joint pain can be helped by nonsteroidal anti-inflammatory drugs. Patients who develop the more severe complications, including progressive renal involvement or severe GI disturbances, have been treated with cyclophosphamide, cylosporin, azathioprine, and plasmaphoresis. Most of the evidence is based on case reports and case series.

The condition is usually self-limiting though the older the patient, the more likely there are to be longer-term complications, particularly renal disease. The renal lesion in Henoch-Schönlein purpura is an immunoglobulin A nephropathy, histologically identical to that seen in Berger's disease. Patients who appear to recover need to be followed up for several months with regular checks of renal function and urine analysis to ensure that later complications are not setting in.

Patient 66

A 91-year-old man fell from the second rung of a ladder onto grass while picking apples. He was unable to rise from the ground due to severe pain in his left leg. He was taken to hospital and at the Accident and Emergency Department was found to have an oblique fracture of the left femoral mid shaft, which was treated operatively with a long plate. Until the injury he had enjoyed excellent health and his only medication was tamsulosin for benign prostatic hypertrophy. He was transferred to a rehabilitation ward on the third postoperative day. At that time, on examination, he was afebrile and was noted to be of slim build. His GCS was 15 and AMTS 9/10. His pulse was 78 bpm and regular, with normal heart sounds and no signs of cardiac failure. BP was 145/85 mmHg. Examination of the chest, abdomen, CNS, and the rest of his skeleto-muscular system was normal or satisfactory within the context of his age. A routine bedside urine test revealed heavy glycosuria but was otherwise normal. His oxygen saturation on breathing air was 98%.

Renal function, electrolytes, thyroid function, and screening liver function tests were all normal. A random blood glucose was 14.6 mmol/L and a fasting blood sugar taken the next day was 9.6 mmol/L (3–6). A chest radiograph and an ECG were both normal. A phone call to his GP revealed no history of diabetes mellitus and at a recent Well Elderly check-up, 3 months earlier, he had a normal full blood count, renal function, ESR, and random blood glucose.

Investigations (normal range)

Haemoglobin of 11.0 g/dL (13–18)
Total white cell count 12.2 × 10^9/L (4–11)
ESR 48 mm/h (<20)

---

1 What is the most likely explanation for his current glucose intolerance?

---

2 The most likely reason for the high total white cell count and ESR is:
   A Sepsis.   D Tamsulosin.
   B Myeloma.   E Trauma.
   C Extreme old age.

---

3 How should the high blood glucose be managed?

---

4 What short-term and long-term prophylactic treatments might be needed?

Patient 67

An 83-year-old retired dockyard worker presented with severe dyspnoea and chest pain. His oxygen saturation on air was 89%. His chest radiograph taken on admission is shown (**67a**).

1 What is the most likely cause of the abnormalities shown?
   A Pneumonia.   D RA.
   B Heart failure.   E Mesothelioma.
   C Nephrotic syndrome.

2 What is the most important immediate management step?
   A Administer diuretics intravenously.
   B Administer diuretics orally.
   C Perform a pleural biopsy.
   D Aspirate the pleural fluid.
   E Intravenous antibiotics with oxygen.

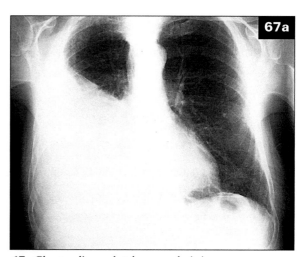

67a Chest radiograph taken on admission.

Patient 66 Answers

1 The patient was known to be in good health with no evidence of diabetes before he fractured his femur. It is known that patients, particularly older people, frequently have glucose intolerance in response to trauma. The mechanism of this has not been fully elucidated but is likely to be due, at least in part, to high levels of cortisol in the post-trauma phase. The hypercortisolaemia tends to persist longer in older people when compared with the young. Of course, it is possible that the patient already had undiagnosed diabetes mellitus and he would certainly need further investigation.

---

2 E Trauma.

The most likely reason for the high total white cell count and moderate rise in ESR is trauma. The mechanism for the high white cell count is probably mainly post-trauma hypercortisolaemia, though that would not explain the high ESR. Patients with large fractures often have a mild to moderate rise in ESR, partly due to the release of acute-phase proteins such as fibrinogen and CRP in response to injury, and possibly also partly due to activation of inflammatory pathways. Both would be expected to fall during the recovery phase, though the hypercortisolaemia can persist for several weeks in some individuals. There is no evidence of sepsis in this case and no reason to suspect myeloma as the ESR and full blood count have been shown to be normal only a few weeks before the injury. Old age would not in itself account for the findings.

3 The glucose intolerance in such a patient might be transient, particularly if it is solely due to the high cortisol levels prevailing after the injury. In such a case it might not be necessary to start any specific treatment, other than to monitor the blood glucose levels until they return to normal. If very high levels occur, the patient will need temporary management with small doses of insulin or an oral antihyperglycaemic agent. If the glucose intolerance persists, and particularly if the cortisol levels have been shown to have returned to normal, the patient is likely to require longer-term management of a diabetic state. The choice of therapy depends on the pattern of the illness, the patient's weight and lifestyle, and other co-morbidities.

4 A patient with a long plate for a mid femoral shaft fracture will be relatively immobile for 3–4 weeks, though partial weight-bearing can be started relatively early. There is a substantial risk of DVT for which mechanical prophylaxis with graduated compression stockings would be sensible. Patients who are more immobile require thromboprophylaxis with low-molecular weight heparin, once perioperative haemostasis has been achieved. The most important long-term prophylactic measure in this patient would be to give a bisphosphonate, calcium, and vitamin D to try to improve tensile bone strength. The patient's fracture occurred after a relatively low energy impact (short fall onto a grassy surface) so he is very likely to be osteoporotic.

Patient 67 Answers

---

1 E Mesothelioma.

---

2 D Aspirate the pleural fluid.

The radiograph shows a large pleural effusion on the right side. In addition, there is pleural calcification above the left diaphragm and pleural thickening along the left hemi thorax. These radiological findings coupled with the history of being a dockyard worker (risk of exposure to asbestos) make mesothelioma the most likely cause of the abnormalities.

This patient presents with severe shortness of breath. The most immediate aim of management would be symptom relief, and aspiration of the pleural fluid is a priority. There is no evidence of heart failure or pneumonia in this patient, therefore diuretics or antibiotics will not offer significant symptom relief. The process of obtaining a histological diagnosis can wait until the patient is symptomatically better.

67b Chest
radiograph
showing
pleural
plaques.

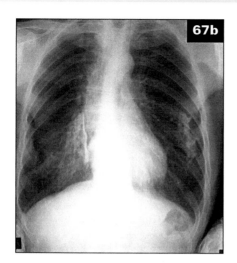

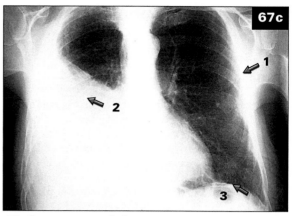

67c Consequences of asbestos exposure. 1, pleural
thickening; 2, pleural effusion; 3, pleural calcification.

Tutorial (Patient 67)

It is generally accepted that mesothelioma is almost always associated with asbestos exposure. Blue asbestos is the usual causative agent. The illness often develops 20–40 years after exposure. Apart from mesothelioma, asbestos may also cause pulmonary fibrosis, squamous carcinoma of the lung, and pleural plaques (**67b, 67c**). Plaques are indicative of exposure and are not in themselves premalignant, although patients who have plaques are more likely to develop other asbestos related illnesses. This may generate anxiety and this has been recognized in a recent court ruling as an adverse outcome of asbestos exposure. Patients may be entitled to compensation for the presence of plaques.

Patient 68

A 73-year-old man presented with an inability to walk. He complained of right foot pain (**68**). He denied any trauma. He had a past history of hypertension and was taking aspirin 75 mg daily, frusemide 40 mg daily, and amlodipine 5 mg daily, and had started taking allopurinol for hand tophi and hyperuricaemia 2 weeks ago. He was on no other medication.

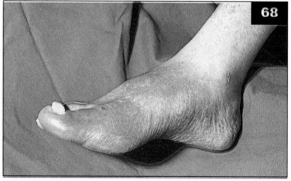

68 Painful right foot.

1 What is the most likely reason for the onset of his symptoms?
 A Cellulitis.
 B Deep vein thrombosis.
 C Allopurinol therapy.
 D Aspirin sensitivity.
 E Metatarsal stress fracture.

2 What test would be most useful to help confirm the diagnosis?
 A Serum uric acid.
 B Polarized microscopy of joint fluid.
 C Radiograph of the foot.
 D Sono-venogram of the foot.
 E Urinalysis and microscopy.

Patient 68 Answers

1 C Allopurinol therapy.

2 B Polarized microscopy of joint fluid.

The appearance of the foot with erythema around the metatarso-phalyngeal joint of the big toe suggests acute gout. This is a well-known complication after starting allopurinol therapy. Prophylaxis is needed when commencing allopurinol and this needs to be continued for some months, even after serum urate levels have returned to normal. NSAIDs are usually given for prophylaxis though colchicine is sometimes preferred for this purpose, being cheaper and well tolerated, especially in patients with peptic ulcer, GI bleeding or dyspepsia, or who are taking anticoagulants.

The history is important and can lead to a working diagnosis in many cases. Gout usually presents in one joint at a time, while other arthritic conditions, such as systemic lupus and RA, usually involve multiple joints simultaneously. Blood tests may support the diagnosis by showing high urate levels, but these levels are also sometimes elevated in the absence of gout, and in this patient hyperuricaemia had already been confirmed. In addition, the uric acid in the blood may be normal in some cases of acute gout. The diagnosis is made if negatively birefringent needle-shaped urate crystals are seen in the joint aspirate when examined under polarized light by microscope. A radiograph of the foot is not likely to show abnormalities apart from soft tissue swelling in early cases of gout. A sono-venogram is not indicated in this case.

Tutorial

First attacks of gout commonly occur in men aged 30–60 years. At first presentation it affects the metatarso-phalyngeal joint of the big toe, a condition known as podagra; in most cases, though other peripheral joints can be affected. It rarely occurs in the axial skeleton or large joints such as the hip or shoulder (and almost never as the first site). It can also present as tenosynovitis, bursitis, or cellulitis. The initial attack can be sudden, waking the patient from sleep. The affected joint becomes red, hot and swollen, with shiny skin. It is very tender and painful. Attacks may be accompanied by fever, leukocytosis and raised erythrocyte sedimentation rate, and preceded by prodromal symptoms. Untreated attacks last days to weeks and are self-limiting. The later stages of gout are decribed on page 120. *Table 68* presents the risk factors for gout.

Table 68 *Risk factors and triggers for gout*

Risk factors
- Genetic predisposition for an abnormality in handling urate accounts for approximately half of all cases. A family history of gout can be a risk factor
- Men of middle age
- High BP
- Drugs:
  - Cytoxics
  - Thiazides
  - Frusemide
  - Ethambutol
  - Salicylates in low dosage
  - Pyrazinamide
  - Sulphonamides
- Obesity or excessive weight gain, especially in youth
- Moderate to heavy alcohol intake
- Abnormal renal function
- Western lifestyle
- Underlying diseases with a high turnover of cells (malignancy, especially blood neoplasms, and haemolytic anaemia)

Triggers
- Recent surgery
- Dehydration
- Joint injury
- Excessive dining
- Heavy alcohol intake (particularly beer, that has a high purine content)
- Stress
- Change in diet
- Certain high purine foods such as red meat and shellfish

Patient 69

An 86-year-old woman who lived alone was admitted after being found collapsed by neighbours. She denied alcohol abuse. She had a BMI of 23 kg/m². She had spontaneous bleeding from the gums, which were also noted to be of abnormal appearance (**69a**). She also had extensive bruising of the legs (**69b**) but the rest of the physical examination was normal.

Her basic liver function tests were normal. Vitamin K corrected the INR but the bleeding persisted and her haemoglobin dropped to 6.5 g/dL. A gastroscopy and colonoscopy were normal.

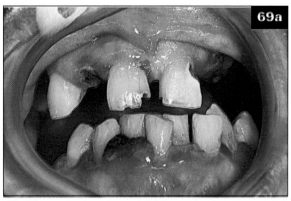

69a The patient's gums at initial examination.

69b The appearance of the legs.

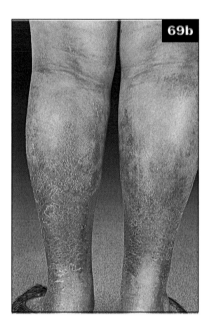

Investigations (normal range)

Haemoglobin 8.9 g/dL (11.5–16.5)
Total white cell count 4.5 × 10⁹/L (4–11)
Platelet count 150 × 10⁹/L (150–400)
Serum folate 0.8 µm/IL (1.7–13.0)
Red cell folate 85 µm/L (85–500)
Plasma fibrinogen 2.5 g/L (1.5–4.0)
Thrombin time 13 s (12–16)
INR 1.9
APTT 27 s (26–40)

---

1 What is the most likely cause of the bleeding?
  A Alcoholic liver cirrhosis.
  B Myelodysplasia.
  C Folate deficiency.
  D Scurvy.
  E Disseminated intravascular coagulation.

Patient 70

A 91-year-old man was found to be dehydrated after spending 2 days on the floor of his flat. He was agitated and it proved difficult to maintain an intravenous line. A decision was made to give subcutaneous fluids.

1 Which of these fluids can be safely administered subcutaneously?
  A Hartman's solution.
  B 10% dextrose.
  C 0.9% saline.
  D Fresh frozen plasma.
  E Sterile water.

Patient 69 Answer

1 D Scurvy.

The spontaneous bleeding offers a wide differential diagnosis. Despite a normal BMI this woman showed evidence of multiple vitamin deficiencies. The bleeding persisted after correction of her INR with vitamin K. In the presence of normal platelets and a normal oesophagogastro-duodenoscopy and colonoscopy, an acquired vascular abnormality is likely. Scurvy is the most likely diagnosis in this case. The gums show gingival hyperplasia. Folic acid deficiency can occur in scurvy due to lack of protection of folate co-enzymes that maintain body folate in the reduced active state. There is no evidence to support a diagnosis of alcoholic liver cirrhosis, myelodysplasia, or disseminated intravascular coagulation; in the last a low platelet count and fibrinogen level would be expected.

Tutorial

The human body is unable to synthesise vitamin C and a diet deficient in vitamin C results in scurvy. Adult scurvy is common in elderly people living alone who prepare their own food or who have particular food fads. Alcoholism, smoking, acute illness, and GI disease all predispose to scurvy.

Vitamin C is a co-factor in the synthesis of collagen and deficiency leads to the breakdown of connective tissue in and around blood vessels and other structures. This leads to manifestations such as the corkscrew appearance of hair follicles and spontaneous bleeding. Scurvy can mimic disorders such as vasculitis, systemic bleeding disorders, and deep vein thrombosis. Typically, vitamin C deficiency is not isolated and other nutritional deficiencies should be sought.

Vitamin C deficiency is diagnosed by the Vitamin C Saturation Test or by measuring leukocyte or serum ascorbic acid levels. Plasma vitamin C is nearly always undetectable in patients with overt scurvy but the range in healthy subjects is too variable for it to be of diagnostic value. Probably the best test to make the diagnosis is still the Vitamin C Saturation Test as it has been shown that leukocyte vitamin C levels may not identify all patients. Prognosis is excellent and clinical improvement is usually apparent soon after starting vitamin C supplements.

Patient 70 Answer

1 C 0.9% saline.

Approximately 3 L of fluid can be given subcutaneously in a 24-hour period at two separate sites. Common infusion sites are the chest, abdomen, thighs, and upper arms. The preferred solution is normal saline, but other solutions, such as half-normal saline, glucose with saline, or 5% glucose, can also be used. Concern has been expressed that the rapid subcutaneous infusion of electrolyte-free solution can cause hypotension. Shock has been reported with the subcutaneous infusion of 5% dextrose in children and 10% dextrose in adults. Several authors have, however, reported the safe administration of 5% dextrose subcutaneously and careful administration of small amounts is safe. This is important as hypertonic dehydration is common in the elderly. Potassium chloride has also been added to the solution bag when needed. There are reports that this may lead to subcutaneous inflammation. In view of such conflicting information some local policies may preclude giving 5% dextrose or potassium chloride subcutaneously. It is important therefore to check with local guidelines before administering such fluids. Hyaluronidase can also be added to enhance fluid absorption. This is useful when one wishes to administer a relatively large volume of fluid at a single site.

Fluids can be given as a continuous infusion throughout a 24-hour period, as an overnight infusion, or a rapid intermittent infusion of up to 500 ml of fluid over 20 minutes. In general, however, no more than 3 L should be administered over a 24-hour period. It may be difficult to give more than 1.5 L at a single site. Because of the risk of hypotension, no more than 2 L of 5% dextrose should be administered subcutaneously over 24 hours with a maximim of 2 ml/minute at any one time.

Patient 71

A 75-year-old patient with general joint pains was noted to have the rash shown in Figure 71.

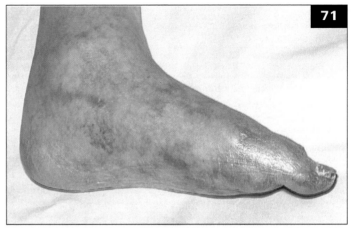

71 The patient's foot, showing skin rash.

1 What is this rash?
  A Livedo reticularis.
  B Cutis marmorata.
  C Erythema ab igne.
  D Erythema nodosum.
  E Erythema marginatum.

Patient 72

A 67-year-old man presented with a dry cough and a 2-year history of shortness of breath and weight loss. Physical examination revealed hard lumps around his fingers. He looked cyanosed and his PaO$_2$ was 7.5 kPa (11.3–12.6). He had normal spirometry.

A plain radiograph of his hands is shown in Figure 72.

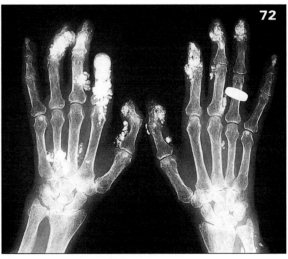

72 Plain radiograph of the hands.

1 What is the most likely cause of this patient's cyanosis?
  A Pneumonia.
  B Pulmonary fibrosis.
  C Pulmonary vascular disease.
  D Adult-onset asthma.
  E COPD.

Patient 71 Answer

> 1 A Livedo reticularis.

The rash is livedo reticularis. Livedo reticularis refers to a condition in which dilatation of capillary blood vessels and stagnation of blood within them causes a mottled discolouration of the skin. It is described as being a reticular (net-like), cyanotic (reddish blue), cutaneous discolouration surrounding pale central areas. It occurs mostly on the legs, arms, and trunk and is more pronounced in cold weather. *Table 71* presents the causes.

Cutis marmorata causes temporary livedo in about 50% of normal infants and many children and adults when exposed to the cold and is a physiological response. Erythema ab igne is a reticular pigmented rash that develops after chronically exposing a part of the body to a hot or warm object, such as a hot water bottle. Erythema nodosum consists of red tender raised areas of skin mostly on the extensor surfaces of the legs and arms. Erythema marginatum consists of pink coalescing rings usually on the trunk that come and go.

Table 71 *Causes of livedo reticularis*

Idiopathic
Mostly in young and middle aged females, particularly during winter; occurs on exposure to cold

Secondary causes:
Vasculitis
- Livedoid vasculitis
- Polyarteritis nodosa
- SLE
- Dermatomyositis
- RA
- Lymphoma
- Pancreatitis
- TB

Obstruction
- Cryoglobulinaemia (immunoglobulins that precipitate in the cold)
- Antiphospholipid syndrome or lupus anticoagulant syndrome
- Hypercalcaemia
- Polycythaemia rubra vera (excessive number of red cells) or thrombocythaemia (platelet clumps)
- Infections (syphilis, TB)
- Arteriosclerosis (cholesterol emboli) and homocystinuria
- Intra-arterial injection in drug addicts

Patient 72 Answer

> 1 C Pulmonary vascular disease.

The most likely cause for his symptoms and cyanosis is pulmonary vascular disease associated with systemic sclerosis. The normal spirometry makes pulmonary fibrosis much less likely. Age at the onset of scleroderma is an important risk factor for PAH. There is a twofold greater risk of PAH for late-onset (age 60 years) versus earlier-onset (<60 years) disease. Vigilance of these high-risk patients may provide an opportunity to intervene prior to development of irreversible pulmonary vascular disease.

Tutorial

Scleroderma is an unusual form of connective tissue disorder, literally translated as 'hardening of the skin'. There are two major forms, systemic and localized. Systemic forms of scleroderma occur in two patterns – diffuse systemic sclerosis and limited systemic sclerosis. The former consists of scleroderma with more generalized skin involvement as well as involvement of other systems, particularly the oesophagus, joints, intestines, lungs, heart, and kidneys. It varies greatly in severity and in the rate of progression of the disease. It can range from the widespread thickening of skin (diffuse) to a form with more limited skin involvement (CREST).

CREST is an acronym made up of the first letters of the five most prominent manifestations of this form of scleroderma:
Calcinosis (due to deposition of calcium salts under the skin)
Raynaud's phenonemon
(O) Esophageal dysfunction (the loss of normal action in the lower oesophagus)
Sclerodactyly (hardening of the skin on the digits)
Telangiectasia

The localized forms of scleroderma include morphea, a localized scleroderma which begins with an inflammatory stage followed by the appearance of one or more patches or plaques, and linear scleroderma, which is a band of thickening of the skin often limited to one area.

Patient 73

A 70-year-old patient with sero-positive RA presented unable to walk. Physical examination revealed grade 3/5 weakness of dorsiflexion of the right foot. The plantar reflex was equivocal.

1 Which of the following statements best applies to this case presentation?
  A This may be due to mononeuritis.
  B Rheumatoid factor is undetectable in the patient's serum.
  C Peripheral neuropathy would present with bilateral foot drop.
  D Ischaemic stroke can be safely excluded.
  E Magnetic resonance imaging of the cervical spine is not indicated.

Patient 74

A 70-year-old man presented to the Day Hospital because of increasing difficulty with using his hands. He had a long-standing history of hand pain. Physical examination revealed markedly abnormal hands (**74**).

1 What is the diagnosis?
  A RA.
  B Arthritis mutilans.
  C Erosive OA.
  D Chronic tophaceous gout.
  E Psoriatic arthropathy.

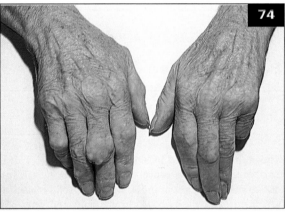

74 Painful abnormal hands.

Patient 75

An 84-year-old man who lived alone was referred with poor mobility. Physical examination revealed a rather unkempt man with severe onychogryphosis.

1 Who was the best person to deal with this condition?
  A Reflexologist.
  B Geriatrician.
  C Nurse specialist.
  D Physiotherapist.
  E Chiropodist.

Patient 73 Answer

---

1 **A** This may be due to mononeuritis.

In sero-positive RA, rheumatoid factor is detectable in the patients serum. Rheumatoid factor is a specific IgM antibody directed against a patient's own IgG antigen. It is synthesized in plasma cells within the synovium of affected joints. It is not possible to come to a definitive single diagnosis on this patient from the limited information above. The weakness of dorsiflexion in this patient with rheumatoid disease suggests a peripheral neuropathy or a mononeuritis. At this age it could also be a stroke or cervical myelopathy associated with rheumatoid disease. The equivocal plantar is unhelpful in differentiating between the possible diagnoses.

Tutorial

RA presents in several ways. Most patients present with insidious multiple joint involvement. There are usually several exacerbations and remissions with variable degrees of functional disability. Some elderly patients present with Sjögren's syndrome and limited joint disease of a benign nature. Others can present with the sudden onset of severe stiffness affecting mostly the large joints. In these patients, who are predominantly male, the disease has very acute onset but a good prognosis, with remission usual within 1 year.

RA is a systemic disease and there is multi system involvement in which almost any organ system can be affected. Manifestations of multi system disease include vasculitis, pericarditis, myocarditis or endocarditis, pleurisy and other pulmonary conditions, renal disease, and neuropathies.

Patient 74 Answer

---

1 **D** Chronic tophaceous gout.

The photograph shows bilateral tophaceous gout. This is associated with progressive cartilage and bone erosion due to the deposition of tophi, which are solid masses of uric acid. These can be seen and palpated over the extensor surfaces of joints and can cause joint erosions, secondary OA and, as in this case, disability caused by permanent restriction of joint function. The patient's function could improve with regular exercise, physiotherapy, and occupational therapy. Adaptive living support would also be needed in such a severe case. The tophi slowly resolve after the serum urate is rendered normal by treatment with allopurinol; this can take 2 years or more.

Tutorial

The natural history of gout has four stages:
- Asymptomatic initial stage characterized with hyperuricaemia. It is important to note that not all hyperuricaemic patients go on to develop gout.
- Acute gouty arthritis. Acute gout most commonly involves the first metatarsal phalangeal joint (known as podagra).
- Intercritical gout (variable symptom-free periods between acute attacks that may last weeks or years).
- Chronic tophaceous gout. Recurrent acute attacks lead to chronic tophaceous gout. This is characterized by progressive cartilage and bone erosion and deposition of tophi (solid masses of uric acid). Patients may develop renal tract stones from high urinary uric acid. The usual sites of tophi are: the helix of the ear, the extensor surfaces of joints, olecranon bursae and, sometimes, in the finger pads. Erosive tophaceous arthritis of the interphalangeal joints of the hands may be mistaken for erosive OA. Gout is usually asymmetrical.

The risk factors for gout are presented in *Table 68* on page 114.

Patient 75 Answer

---

1 **E** Chiropodist.

A chiropodist is the professional who would be best trained to deal with this condition.

Tutorial (Patient 75)

Onychogryphosis is a nail condition characterized by gross thickening and curving of the nails. The disorder usually affects the big toe nail, which becomes greatly thickened and distorted. It is usually seen in elderly patients who find it hard to take care of their feet. It is probably caused by trauma to the nail bed, such as dropping a heavy object onto the toe or more gradual trauma from the toe nail impacting on the inside of the shoe. Nail cutting with conventional clippers becomes nearly impossible. Treatment is by having regular chiropody with grinding of the nail at regular intervals. Surgical removal of the nail and ablation of the nail bed might also be required.

Patient 76

An 80-year-old man complained of recurrent episodes of painful swelling of the right knee. Physical examination revealed a knee effusion and a low-grade temperature. His knee radiograph is shown (**76a**).

76a Plain radiograph of right knee joint.

1 What is the likely diagnosis?
  A Gout.
  B Pyrophosphate arthropathy.
  C Septic arthritis.
  D Psoriatic arthropathy.
  E Reactive arthritis.

Patient 77

A 76-year-old man complained of swelling of his nose (**77**).

77 Lateral view of the nose.

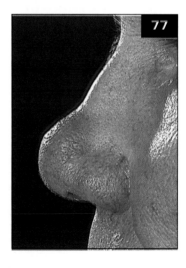

1 Which of the following is his condition most likely to be associated with?
  A Acne rosacea.
  B Acne vulgaris.
  C Psoriasis.
  D Eczema.
  E Sarcoidosis.

Patient 76 Answer

1 **B** Pyrophosphate arthropathy.

The mode of presentation of this patient together with the radiological appearance suggests the diagnosis of pyrophosphate arthropathy (pseudo-gout). Pseudo-gout is one of a spectrum of illnesses caused by deposition of calcium pyrophosphate. The radiograph shows chondro-calcinosis. Chondrocalcinosis is the streaking of cartilage with calcium. It is often associated with pyrophosphate arthropathy. The radiograph shows calcification of the cartilage of the knee (**76b**, arrows). Chondrocalcinosis commonly affects the knees, pubic symphysis, and wrists, but may also involve other joints. Conditions causing chondrocalcinosis are presented in *Table 76*.

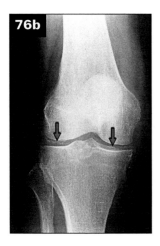

76b Arrows indicate chondrocalcinosis.

Tutorial

Gout can be distinguished from pseudo-gout on light microscopy. In gout the crystals (sodium urate) are needle-shaped and are negative birefringent in polarized light, while pseudo-gout crystals (calcium pyrophosphate) are rhomboid-shaped and have weak positive birefringence. The onset of pseudo-gout is usually monoarticular or pauciarticular, and is often preceded by injury or surgery to the area. It can also follow a parathyroid adenoma excision. It presents in a crescendo reaching a peak in hours, and creating pain, swelling, heat, and redness. Fever is present in approximately half of patients. The CRP is often acutely raised. The knee is the joint most often affected. The shoulder, elbow, ankle, and first MTP joint are also commonly involved.

The natural course is spontaneous resolution over a few days or, at most, weeks. The calcium pyro-phosphate can be deposited in large accumulations at joint margins, producing a pseudo-tumour. This is referred to as tophaceous pseudo-gout. Treatment depends on the severity of signs and symptoms, but may include: injections of corticosteroids directly into the joint; NSAIDs; and prednisolone or colchicine for flares of pseudo-gout.

Table 76 *Conditions causing chondrocalcinosis*

- Hyperparathyroidism
- Haemochromatosis
- Hypophosphatasia
- Hypomagnesaemia
- Wilson's disease
- OA
- Diabetes

Patient 77 Answer

1 **A** Acne rosacea.

This patient has hypertrophy of the sebaceous tissue known as rhinophyma. It results from long-standing acne rosacea.

Tutorial

Acne rosacea is a common skin rash of adults, and becomes commoner with age. There are three stages to the condition. In the first stage the face becomes red. The redness often persists after cold exposure or after exposure to irritants like soap. It may be associated with stinging or burning. In the second stage of rosacea, the redness covers a larger area of the face. Slight swelling, pimples, and pustules develop. This is especially noticeable on the nose, mid forehead, and chin. As the condition progresses, prominent facial pores can develop. The third stage is characterized by swelling and growth of the nose (rhinophyma) and central facial areas. At times the ears may be involved as well. This can be very disfiguring. Most patients do not progress to the third stage of rosacea. The cause is unknown although sunlight may be a factor. Food and beverages causing facial flushing such as alcohol or spicy foods can make the condition appear worse.

Patient 78

An 85-year-old bed-bound woman was noted to have a sacral pressure sore as shown (**78**).

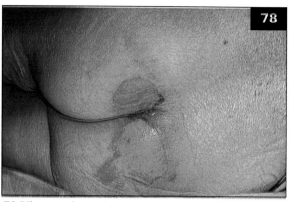

78 Ulcers on buttocks.

1 How would you classify the lesion?
  A Grade 1.
  B Grade 2.
  C Grade 3.
  D Grade 4.
  E Grade 5.

Patient 79

An 85-year-old woman presented with a 6-week history of a rash (**79**) and feeling unwell. She had a history of osteoporosis, ischaemic heart disease, and noninsulin-dependent diabetes. She was a life long nonsmoker and did not drink alcohol. She was not taking any medication that could have precipitated the rash. On examination there were erythematous lesions on the flexor surfaces of the upper limbs, back, and thighs. There was no mucous membrane involvement.

An abdominal ultrasound scan at this stage was normal. Despite successful treatment of her rash she deteriorated over the subsequent 3 months, losing weight and becoming clinically jaundiced.

A repeat ultrasound showed prominent dilatation of the intrahepatic ducts, common bile duct, and pancreatic ducts.

Investigations (normal range)

Serum alkaline phosphatase 606 U/L (30–100)
Serum gamma glutamyl aminotransferase 217 U/L (1–70).
Serum total bilirubin, ALT, albumin, INR, hepatitis serology, and autoantibody screen normal

Subsequent investigations (normal range)
Serum alkaline phosphatase 3020 U/L (30–100)
Serum gamma glutamyl aminotransferase 1904 U/L (1–70)
Serum ALT 211 U/L (7–30)
Serum total bilirubin 141 mmol/L (0–17)

1 What is the rash and how would you confirm the diagnosis?

2 What is the usual treatment of this condition?

3 How would you investigate further the abnormal liver function tests and how might they be related to the rash?

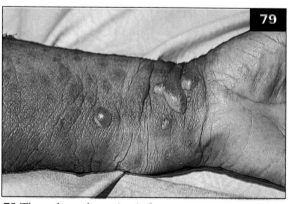

79 The rash on the patient's forearms.

Patient 78 Answer

> **1** B Grade 2.

Figure 78 shows a grade 2 pressure sore. Sores are usually graded according to a classification suggested by the National Pressure Ulcer Advisory Panel (see Patient 21, page 37 for the basic grade definitions). This is a grade 2 pressure sore because there is a partial thickness skin loss involving the epidermis, dermis, or both. Grade 2 is usually a superficial ulcer presenting clinically as an abrasion, blister or shallow crater. The National Pressure Ulcer Advisory Panel classification does not include a grade 5.

Tutorial

A pressure (decubitus) ulcer is a lesion caused by unrelieved pressure, usually over a bony prominence. The incidence in hospitalized patients varies from 2.7% to 29.5% of patients. It is highest in older patients, peaking between the ages of 70 and 80 years. Pressure sores are commonest in the sacral area (40%) followed by the heels (20%), ischial tuberosities (15%), and hips (10%). Other less commonly affected sites include the occiput, ear lobes, elbows, chin, knees, and scapulae. The risk factors for pressure sore development are summarized in *Table 21*.

Unrelieved pressure is the most essential requirement for ulcer development. Perfusion pressures in the arterioles, capillaries, and venules are about 32, 20, and 12 mmHg respectively. Pressure under the ischial tuberosities in a seated position can reach 300 mmHg and sacral pressure can reach 150 mmHg on a standard hospital mattress. Excess pressure results in occlusion of capillary blood flow. Muscle is more easily damaged than skin and is damaged by pressures exceeding mean capillary perfusion pressure for more than an hour.

The mainstay of management is prevention. On the basis of risk factors various scales have been developed. The Braden and Norton Scales are recommended tools in North American Guidelines, while in the UK the Waterlow and Norton scales are the two scales most commonly used. These risk assessment scales however, are based on expert opinion or literature review. Their sensitivity and specificity vary and their effectiveness is limited. Their widespread use often leads to inefficient allocation of preventive measures and there is a need for more accurate risk assessment tools. There is no substitute for medical and nursing vigilance in this context.

Patient 79 Answers

1 The rash was bullous pemphigoid. The diagnosis was confirmed by performing a skin biopsy. It showed eosinophilic micrabscesses in the dermal papillae with an oedematous dermis infiltrated by mild perivascular chronic inflammatory cells. Direct immunoflourescence showed linear deposits of C3 and IgG at the dermo-epidermal junction. Immunology showed positive antibasement membrane antibodies, but negative antidesmosome antibodies confirming a diagnosis of bullous pemphigoid (compare this with the case of pemphigus on page 67).

2 High-dose corticosteroid is the usual treatment.

3 The next investigation would be an ERCP. This suggested the diagnosis of a hilar cholangio-carcinoma. A stent was inserted to treat the obstructive jaundice but there was only a short-term improvement. The final diagnosis was one of bullous pemphigoid as a paraneoplastic presentaion of a cholangio-carcinoma.

Tutorial

Cholangio-carcinoma is a rare tumour accounting for about 10% of primary hepatic tumours with around 400 cases diagnosed per year in the UK. Pemphigoid is similarly an uncommon condition occurring in 1.8/100,000 of the UK population. The occurrence of these two rare conditions together suggests that the pemphigoid was a paraneoplastic manifestation of the cholangio-carcinoma. There is increasing evidence that in elderly patients bullous pemphigoid is associated with internal malignancy, including renal cell carcinoma and non-Hodgkins lymphoma.

Patient 80

A 75-year-old woman presented to the Outpatient Clinic complaining of long-standing lancinating headaches above the right eye with no obvious precipitating or relieving factors. The patient's forehead is shown in Figure **80**. The skin was sensitive to touch but the rest of her physical examination was unremarkable.

1 What is the likely cause of the headaches?
   A Cluster headaches.
   B Tension headaches.
   C Trigeminal neuralgia.
   D Temporal arteritis.
   E Postherpetic neuralgia.

2 Which of these is of no use in treating patients with this condition?
   A Capsaicin cream.
   B Varivax (varicella zoster vaccine).
   C Lignocaine skin patches.
   D TENS.
   E Lamotrigine.

Investigations showed a normal full blood count and an ESR of 50 mm/h.

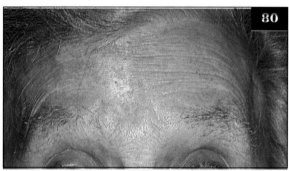

80 The appearance of the patient's forehead.

Patient 81

A 78-year-old woman was admitted with a headache. She gave a past history of ischaemic heart disease and hypertension. On clinical examination she had a left hemi-paresis compli-cating a cerebral haemorrhage. Photographs of her axilla and chest wall are shown (**81a, 81b**).

1 What are the abnormalities identified in the figures?

2 What is the most likely diagnosis?
   A Cachexia.
   B Pseudo-xanthoma elasticum.
   C Tylosis.
   D Acanthosis nigricans.
   E Urticaria.

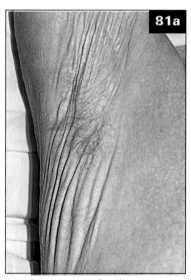

81a Appearance of axilla.

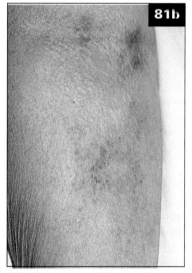

81b Appearance of chest wall.

Patient 80 Answers

1 E Postherpetic neuralgia.

This woman has postherpetic neuralgia. The picture shows scarring of the right side of the forehead with sparing of the left side. This is postherpetic scarring of the skin due to a previous herpes zoster infection. Although the ESR is mildly elevated, it is a nonspecific finding. The headache of temporal arteritis is typically associated with temporal artery tenderness. The presentation of this woman is not suggestive of cluster headaches, tension headaches, or trigeminal neuralgia.

2 B Varivax (varicella zoster vaccine).

The pain is neuropathic and results from abnormal firing of peripheral sensory (nociceptor) neurons. No benefit will result from immunization. Treatment for postherpetic neuralgia also depends on the severity of the pain. Topical treatments can be helpful. Lignocaine skin patches can provide some relief but should not be used long-term on the face as this may cause hypersensitivity. Capsaicin is a cream, made from the seeds of chilli peppers, and can relieve skin pain. It depletes tissues of substance P, which is involved in nociceptor activation. It can cause a burning sensation in the initial stages of treatment and irritates the skin, particularly if rubbed on unaffected skin.

Antidepressants modulate key brain neurotransmitters, including serotonin and noradrenaline. These play a role in both depression and pain mediation. The dose of antidepressant for postherpetic neuralgia is smaller than that used for depression. Tricyclic antidepressants, including amitriptyline do not eliminate the pain but appear to alter the pain threshold, making it easier to

tolerate the symptom. Other antidepressants that can be used include venlafaxine, and SSRIs such as sertraline, paroxetine, and fluoxetine.

Anticonvulsants such as phenytoin can also lessen postherpetic neuralgia by stabilizing cell membranes in injured nerves. Medications such as carbamazepine (particularly for sharp, jabbing pain), gabapentin, and lamotrigine can help control burning sensations and pain.

When the pain is very severe analgesics such as tramadol or fentanyl might need to be used, or even morphine. TENS may be of benefit. Exactly how the impulses relieve pain is uncertain. One theory is that the impulses stimulate production of endorphins.

Tutorial

Postherpetic neuralgia is a painful condition complicating shingles. The varicella zoster virus remains dormant in sensory nerve ganglia after an attack of chickenpox but may be reactivated when age and/or illness and/or medications cause immune suppression (particularly cell-mediated immunity). It can also reactivate for no apparent reason. The incidence of postherpetic neuralgia increases with age. It results from sensory nerve fibre damage during the episode of shingles. In some cases, treatment of postherpetic neuralgia brings complete pain relief. However, most people still experience some pain, and a few have severe continuing pain. Although some people must live with postherpetic neuralgia for the rest of their lives, the majority can expect the condition gradually to disappear within 5 years. Some patients become depressed by the chronic pain and require treatment for depression.

Patient 81 Answers

1 Figure **81a** shows excessive axillary skin folds. Figure **81b** shows the characteristic plucked chicken appearance of the skin. This is due to the presence of numerous small yellow plaques. Skin bruising due to hyper-elasticity and fragility of the skin can also be seen.

2 B Pseudo-xanthoma elasticum.

The diagnosis is PXE. This is an hereditary disorder of connective tissue leading to degeneration of elastic fibres. There are four recognized variants of the condition, two inherited as autosomal dominant and two inherited as autosomal recessive. It presents with multi system manifestations. Often there is ocular, dermal, and cardiovascular involvement. The patient is clearly not thin enough for cachexia to be the cause of the folding, and that condition would not cause the skin to have the 'plucked chicken' texture. Tylosis is an inherited tendency to severe thickening of the skin of the palms and soles. Acanthosis nigricans in the axillae has a pigmented velvety appearance and is often associated with malignant tumours of the oesophagus, stomach, and other foregut structures.

Tutorial (Patient 81)

Cardiovascular manifestations of PXE include premature coronary heart disease, mitral valve prolapse, rupture of the aortic valve, atrial septal aneurysms, hypertension, and peripheral vascular disease. Treatment of cardiovascular complications is problematic. Coronary artery arterial bypass grafts tend to calcify prematurely. The incidence of ischaemic stroke is increased due to small vessel disease but treatment with antiplatelet agents can precipitate bleeding, often leading to difficult treatment decisions. Patients with PXE are more likely to have intracranial artery aneurysms but there is no evidence that they are more likely to be symptomatic than similar lesions in other patients.

Patient 82

A 74-year-old woman presented with patchy discolouration of the skin on her feet (**82**).

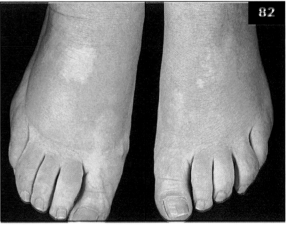

82 Dorsal view of the feet.

1 Which of these conditions is not associated with the above skin condition?
   A Grave's disease.
   B Oesophageal cancer.
   C Alopecia areata.
   D Hashimoto's thyroiditis.
   E Addisons disease.

Patient 83

A 90-year-old female, who lived alone, was admitted to the Accident and Emergency Department on a Friday afternoon with a history of falls. She had a past history of aortic stenosis. Her MMSE score was 22/30. Physical examination revealed an aortic ejection systolic murmur. Her BP was 120/85mmHg with no fall in BP on standing. She was not short of breath and her chest and abdomen were unremarkable. She was frail and had an unsafe 'Get up and Go' Test. In the admissions ward she was noted to manage her ADL with difficulty.

Investigations

Recent echocardiogram showed a peak aortic valve gradient of 28 mmHg with poor left ventricular function
Urinalysis blood + and protein +
Full blood count normal

1 Which of the following is the best management option?
   A Prescribe trimethoprim and discharge home.
   B Discharge to a nursing home.
   C Refer for urgent aortic valve replacement.
   D Refer for physiotherapy and occupational therapy.
   E Discharge and ask her GP to follow-up.

Patient 82 Answer

> **1 B** Oesophageal cancer.

Vitiligo is common, affecting 1 in 100 people. Vitiligo can be found in all parts of the world; it affects all ethnic groups but can be far more disabling in those who have dark skin. There is no association with malignancy.

Tutorial

Vitiligo affects males and females equally. The usual age of onset is between 10 and 30 years old, but the condition can start at any age. A study looked at the clinical and epidemiological profile of vitiligo in the elderly. Vitiligo vulgaris was the commonest (83.5%), followed by focal (5.5%), segmental (4.4%), acrofacial (3.8%), mucosal (2.2%), and universal (0.5%). The most common site of onset was the head and neck (24.2%), followed by the upper limbs (23%), trunk (22%), lower limbs (17.6%), oral/genital mucosae (7.1%), and flexures (6%). Koebner's phenomenon (worsening of the condition caused by local trauma) was observed in 14.8% while leukotrichia was present in 47.3% of the patients. Halo neavi were observed in 3.8% of patients, and vitiligo was stable in 64.8%. Only 15.9% of patients had a family history of vitiligo. Associated autoimmune/endocrine disorders were present in 21.4% of the patients.

Patient 83 Answer

> **1 D** Refer for physiotherapy and occupational therapy.

This woman has no evidence of sepsis. A UTI is therefore unlikely to be the cause of this patient's falls. She does, however, have poor mobility and could benefit from physiotherapy in a rehabilitation environment. Occupational therapy might improve her ability to manage her ADL. Attention to nutrition could also benefit this patient. Admission to a nursing home without consideration being given to rehabilitation first would not be consistent with good management of the patient. One of the main purposes of geriatric medicine is to keep elderly people living safely in their own home as long as possible. This woman, although frail, might improve with rehabilitation and could then return home safely with external support once her needs have been assessed. She has moderate to severe aortic stenosis. However, the risks of open heart surgery in the very elderly are substantial, with an increased risk of stroke and heart failure and other postoperative complications. Furthermore, she had no symptoms directly attributable to the aortic stenosis. Some very aged patients are treated operatively if they are symptomatic (breathlessness, chest pain, syncope) and there are no other therapeutic options, providing they are fit for major surgery. Such decisions may be difficult in real life and, whenever possible, the decision should be discussed with the patient. The first 24–48 hours are crucial for elderly people discharged home. An adequate care package has to be put in place prior to discharge to minimize the risk of readmission and harm from further falls and injury. General medical practice and other support services are usually limited over the weekend and unless one is sure that the patient will receive the support she needs at home she should not be discharged.

Patient 84

A 73-year-old woman known to have advanced dementia, and who lived with her divorced alcoholic son, was admitted to the Accident and Emergency Department after being found on the floor. She had a history of falls. Physical examination revealed extensive bruising especially over the back (**84**). The possibility of physical abuse with violence was raised by a reliable neighbour.

Investigations (normal range)

Haemoglobin 9.5g/dL (11.5–16.5)
Total white cell count 10.0 × 10⁹/L (4–11)
Platelet count 98 × 10⁹/L (150–400)

1 Which would be the best initial steps in this patient's management?
  A Ignore the possibility of elder abuse as this is not your problem.
  B Admit and send for the patient's son to explain the bruises.
  C Discharge home and refer to social services.
  D Admit to a nursing home and refer to social services.
  E Admit, investigate for possible blood disorders and involve social services and/or the police.

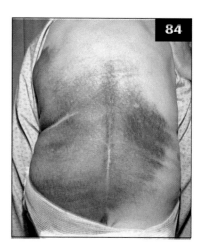

84 The extent of the bruising.

Patient 85

A 68-year-old previously independent patient presented with decreasing mobility, falls, fatigue, and pain in his right leg. Physical examination showed generalized pain on movement of the right leg. The rest of the physical examination was unremarkable. A photograph of the patient's legs is shown (**85**).

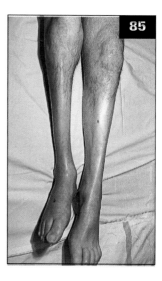

85 The appearance of the patient's legs.

Investigations

Full blood count, serum urea, creatinine, electrolytes, liver screen, thyroid function, and random glucose all normal
Radiographs of the right and left hip showed early osteoarthritic changes but no fractures

1 What childhood illness had the patient suffered from?
  A Congenital dislocation of the hip.
  B Duchenne muscular dystrophy.
  C Poliomyelitis.
  D Rickets.
  E Facioscapulohumoral muscle dystrophy.

2 What is the most likely cause of the patient's current symptoms?
  A Malnutrition.
  B Postpolio syndrome.
  C OA.
  D Hip pain.
  E Leg shortening.

Patient 84 Answer

> 1 E Admit, investigate for possible blood disorders and involve social services and/or the police.

The best option is to admit and involve social services and/or the police. This woman would also need investigation of her anaemia and thrombocytopenia. However, with extensive bruising such as this, a crime could possibly have been committed and the police or social services would want to be involved as soon as possible as investigation of a possible crime scene might be required. Ignoring the possibility of elder abuse in this vulnerable adult is negligent and discharging home is not to be considered at this stage. Discharging to a nursing home with social services input is not the best option at this stage and is premature. There are still unresolved issues as to how best to deal with the thrombocytopenia.

Tutorial

In this situation the patient is a vulnerable adult with lack of capacity so decisions have to be taken on her behalf and in her best interests by the health care professionals looking after her. It is permitted to break patient confidentiality if the patient is at risk, or has a notifiable disease, and/or is thought to be an active threat to public safety.

Patient 85 Answers

> 1 C Poliomyelitis.

> 2 B Postpolio syndrome.

The figure shows that the left leg is smaller and the muscles atrophic, indicating stunted growth of the limb in childhood. The patient had suffered childhood poliomyelitis. Acute poliomyelitis is a viral infection of the anterior horn cells within the spinal cord causing varying degrees of muscle paralysis while sensation remains intact.

The most likely cause for his symptoms is the postpolio syndrome. This is diagnosed in the absence of other significant abnormalities or likely illnesses.

Tutorial

Poliomyelitis damages lower motor neurons with consequent muscle atrophy. The remaining musculature has to function at a higher demand than normal to maintain mobility. Patients usually improve their function through substitution from other muscles and/or by using passive tendon tension by alternate posturing. This introduces the potential for overuse of remaining muscles. The postpolio syndrome is characterized by loss of strength, increased fatigue, and muscle or joint pain. Between 60 and 80% of sufferers develop symptoms, often many years after the initial attack. Polio patients are particularly likely to develop these problems in old age. There is strong experimental evidence demonstrating the loss of muscle fibres through damage from overuse, oedema, inflammatory cell infiltration, and fibre degeneration. Muscle pain is a sign of injury. The key point is that most patients with loss of function are not suffering from inactivity. Exercise can make only a small contribution to the management plan. The primary therapeutic programme is to reduce the strain on the affected muscles by lifestyle modification or assistive equipment. If strain can be relieved, there can be mild improvement of strength and significant improvement of function.

The diagnosis is one of exclusion. Other conditions that have similar symptoms must be ruled out. These include fibromyalgia, multiple sclerosis, myasthenia gravis, Parkinson's disease, tumours, and so on. Having postpolio syndrome obviously does not rule out the possibility of having another disease superimposed. Once the diagnosis is made it needs to be reviewed as new symptoms develop.

Patient 86

A 79-year-old man was referred urgently for rehabilitation several weeks after a left hip replacement. His progress was hampered because of persistent back pain unrelieved by various NSAIDs. He also complained of constipation and insomnia. His pelvic radiograph is shown (**86**).

1 What is *unlikely* to be contributing to his poor progress?
  A Failed hip replacement.
  B OA of hip.
  C Prostatic carcinoma.
  D Faecal overload.
  E OA of the spine.

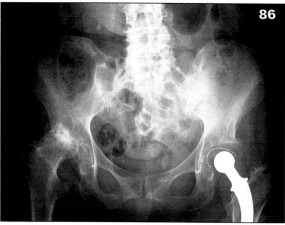

86 Plain radiograph of the pelvis.

Patient 87

A geriatrician was asked to see a very frail bed-bound 89-year-old woman in a nursing home who had recently started vomiting. She had no specific complaints apart from feeling generally unwell and nauseous. She had a past history of atrial fibrillation, OA, and COPD. She was taking digoxin 250 µg daily and ibuprofen 200 mg three times daily. On examination she appeared dehydrated and had a BMI of 15 kg/m² and weighed 45 kg. Her BP was 135/85 mmHg with a pulse of 55 bpm irregular. Her chest and abdomen were unremarkable on examination.

Investigations (normal range)

Haemoglobin 10.5 g/dL (11.5–16.5)
Total white cell count 4.5 × 10⁹/L
Platelet count 155 × 10⁹/L
Serum urea 17.8 mmol/L (2.5–7.5)
Serum sodium 145 mmol/L (137–144)
Serum potassium 4.5 mmol/L (3.5–4.9)
Serum creatinine 155 mmol/L (60–110)

1 How would you first investigate this patient's symptoms?
  A Request a gastroscopy.
  B Measure serum digoxin level.
  C Perform ultrasound of the renal tract.
  D Measure creatinine clearance.
  E Request an ESR.

Patient 88

A 72-year-old retired accountant presented with a dry cough and shortness of breath. He had a past history of ischaemic heart disease and atrial fibrillation, but denied any chest pain. His medication was aspirin 75 mg daily, warfarin, and amiodarone 100 mg daily. His chest radiograph is shown (**88**).

1 What is the most likely diagnosis?
  A Bronchopneumonia.
  B Bronchogenic carcinoma.
  C Mesothelioma.
  D Pulmonary fibrosis.
  E Heart failure.

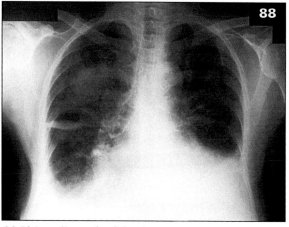

88 Plain radiograph of the chest.

Patient 86 Answer

> **1 A** Failed hip replacement.

This radiograph is very typical of elderly patients undergoing rehabilitation. It demonstrates multiple pathologies, some of which are irreversible due to chronic degenerative disease. The left hip prosthesis is in place and technically the operation was successful. It is therefore unlikely to be causing any significant problems.

Sometimes there may be residual pain and persistent postoperative muscle weakness. These do not seem to be a problem in this man. There is, however, pathology elsewhere. There is significant OA in his right hip and spine. In addition, there is sclerosis of the bones of the lumbar spine suggestive of metastatic disease from a carcinoma of the prostate. There is also evidence of faecal loading. Significant constipation is very common and can have an adverse affect on rehabilitation

Patient 87 Answer

> **1 B** Measure serum digoxin level.

This woman is likely to have digoxin toxicity. Her symptoms and bradycardia are consistent with the diagnosis. She is on a high dose of digoxin for her weight. Her renal function is impaired which would further enhance the risk of toxicity. Checking her digoxin level and reducing the dose is essential.

This patient's symptoms of nausea and vomiting could be due to upper GI ulceration or gastritis caused by the ibuprofen. However, she is very frail and bed-bound. Invasive investigations such as an OGD can be technically difficult and arguably not in the patient's best interest. A more pragmatic approach to the possibility of upper GI ulceration is required. Changing the ibuprofen to an alternative analgesic and/or prescribing a proton pump inhibitor would be a better treatment approach in this case.

Renal tract ultrasound might be useful in investigating the possible cause of her renal failure. However, the disproportionate rise in urea compared to creatinine suggests dehydration, or possibly GI blood loss, as the cause of her renal failure, therefore an ultrasound is not an important initial investigation. Formal measurement of creatinine clearance is unlikely to add much more information about the patient's clinical condition. Similarly, an ESR is not a very helpful or discriminatory investigation in this clinical context.

Patient 88 Answer

> **1 E** Heart failure.

This patient has heart failure and the chest radiograph shows several features of this condition. There is cardiomegaly with bilateral pleural effusions more prominent on the left. There is fluid in the horizontal fissure on the right and there is patchy shadowing in the right upper/mid zone.

Patient 89

An 86-year-old man presented with a 2-day history of breathlessness and an acute confusional state. He lived in a residential home, was normally able to walk unaided, and was independent in the personal ADL. His recent previous medical history was of hypertension and a suspected TIA, for which he had been taking bendroflumethiazide 2.5 mg daily and aspirin 75 mg daily for the last 4 years. His earlier medical history was unknown. He was a nonsmoker. On examination he was afebrile, disorientated in time and place, and anxious. Pulse was 96 bpm regular, heart sounds normal, JVP normal, BP 140/90 mmHg, respiratory rate 24 per minute with wheezy breathing. Auscultation revealed expiratory rhonchi throughout both lungs and a prolonged expiratory phase during tidal breathing. He was using accessory muscles of respiration. Examination of the abdomen was normal. There were no focal or lateralizing neurological signs and his skeleto-muscular system showed mild osteoarthrotic changes only. Oxygen saturation was 88% on room air and 94% on 28% oxygen.

His chest radiograph is shown (**89**).

> *Investigations (normal range)*
>
> Haemoglobin 13.1 g/dL (11.5–16.5)
> Total white cell count 5.1×10^9/L (4–11)
> Differential white cell count normal
> Serum urea 7.4 mmol/L (2.5–7.5)
> Serum creatinine 74 µmol/L (60–110)
> Serum sodium 140 mmol/L (137–144)
> Serum potassium 3.6 mmol/L (3.5–4.9)
> Arterial PO_2 (breathing air) 8.1 kPa (11.3–12.6)
> Arterial PCO_2 5.1 kPa (4.7–6)
> pH 7.39 (7.36–7.44)

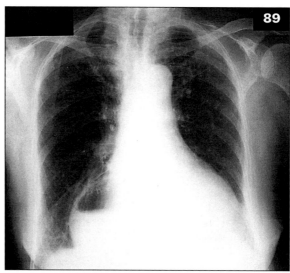

89 Plain radiograph of the chest.

1 What does the chest radiograph show?

2 How might the chest radiograph abnormalities be connected?

3 The next stage of emergency treatment, after oxygen supplementation, is:
   A Antibiotics.
   B Nebulized salbutamol.
   C Proton pump inhibitor.
   D Intravenous aminophylline.
   E Nasogastric tube.

4 How should the patient be further managed and monitored?

5 What long-term treatment might be needed?

Patient 89 Answers

1 The chest radiograph shows hyperinflation of the lungs and a fluid level in a large hiatus hernia. There is probably mild cardiomegaly, though the hiatus hernia shadow, being superimposed on that of the heart shadow, makes it difficult to assess the cardiothoracic ratio.

2 The patient has symptoms and signs of acute diffuse airways obstruction. In a patient without previous known chest disease, this is most likely to be due to asthma. In a majority of patients there would be no clear-cut relationship between asthma and a hiatus hernia. There is some relationship between asthma and gastro-oesophageal reflux, the mechanism of which is uncertain but might be mediated through autonomic reflexes. Also, some patients with a large hiatus hernia aspirate into their airways, though in such cases, the symptoms are more likely to be cough and expectoration, and a chest radiograph could show evidence of aspiration pneumonia. Patients with pulmonary oedema sometimes present with wheezy breathlessness and are mistakenly thought to have asthma. Although the cardiac silhouette is slightly enlarged in this patient, there is no other evidence of pulmonary oedema.

---

3 **B** Nebulized salbutamol.

The patient has evidence of acute diffuse airways obstruction so it would be logical, after giving oxygen, to proceed with a nebulized bronchodilator such as salbutamol. In the majority of patients this will give early improvement of the airflow obstruction with a reduction in the feeling of breathlessness and an improvement in oxygenation. Infection can be a trigger for asthma at any age, and it is quite possible that the patient described above has infection-triggered asthma. However, there is no indication to give an antibiotic as he is afebrile, has a normal white cell count, is not expectorating discoloured sputum, and has no evidence of inflammatory shadowing on the chest radiograph. Infection-triggered asthma is usually caused by viruses such as respiratory syncytial virus. The presence of a large hiatus hernia is not in itself an indication for giving a proton pump inhibitor and, in any case, this patient has no immediate clinical problem requiring that treatment. Intravenous aminophylline can be used as adjunctive therapy in patients with acute diffuse airways obstruction, though it is unusual for it to be used as a first line treatment. There is no indication to pass a nasogastric tube.

4 Having started initial management with oxygen and nebulized salbutamol, the next essential stage is to obtain a chest radiograph to rule out other complicating factors such as a pneumothorax. Unless the patient settles very rapidly on nebulized bronchodilators, it is usual practice to give corticosteroids to suppress airways inflammation and speed recovery. Careful monitoring of the arterial blood gases (or at least oxygen saturation) is required and the patient needs to be observed frequently, using a structured observation chart, to obtain early warning of a deterioration that might require high dependency care. Older patients with asthma become fatigued more rapidly than younger patients and are more likely to require ventilatory support. Once the patient's confusion has settled, the airways obstruction should be monitored by the measurement of peak expiratory flow rate and, if the patient is able to cooperate sufficiently, full spirometry should be obtained at a later stage.

5 Asthma can occur for the first time in old age, though there is often a history of a tendency to wheezing at an earlier stage in life. Nonsmokers presenting with acute diffuse airflow obstruction almost always prove to have asthma as defined by the degree of airways reversibility. Once the acute episode has settled, proper assessment is required and the patient should be considered for long-term maintenance treatment with inhaled bronchodilators and inhaled corticosteroids. Patients with cognitive impairment (particularly if the AMTS is less than 7/10 and/or MMSE score is less than 24/30) are usually unable to learn to use complex inhaler devices. Patients with mild cognitive impairment can sometimes learn to use simple devices such as the Turbohaler. Others with more significant degrees of cognitive impairment will require assistance from another person to use an inhaler (usually with a spacer) or receive supervised treatment by nebulizer. Older patients with asthma often have a poor perception of worsening of their condition, so it is usually advisable to give treatments regularly rather than depend on the patient to use rescue therapy with a fast-acting bronchodilator.

Patient 90

A 75-year-old woman who lived indoors and had a poor diet presented with general aches, worse in the right hip, and persistent vomiting. She was on no regular medication although she took an herbal preparation.

A gastroscopy was normal. A radiograph of her pelvis is shown (**90a**).

Investigations (normal range)

Serum urea 29 mmol/L (2.5–7.5)
Serum creatinine 180 mmol/L (60–110)
Serum sodium and potassium normal
Serum corrected calcium 3.7 mmol/L (2.2–2.6)
Serum phosphate 1.7 mmol/L (0.8–1.4)
Serum alkaline phosphatase 84 U/L (45–105)

1 What is the least useful investigation?
   A Urine for Bence Jones protein.
   B Parathyroid hormone assay.
   C Plasma protein electrophoresis.
   D Chest radiograph.
   E Serum 25-OH Vitamin D.

2 On the basis of the radiograph which diagnosis is the most likely?
   A Hyperparathyroidism.
   B Constipation.
   C Multiple myeloma.
   D Osteomalacia.
   E Sarcoidosis.

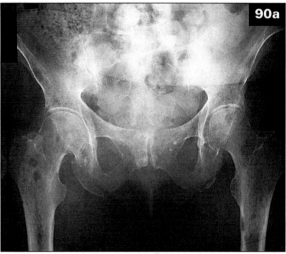

90a Plain radiograph of the pelvis.

Patient 91

An 80-year-old patient was referred to the Outpatient Department by her GP, who found an ESR of 50 mm/h. She was otherwise asymptomatic and rather annoyed at having wasted an afternoon coming to the clinic.

1 Which of the following is the most correct statement?
   A ESR rises with age.
   B This patient is likely to have myeloma.
   C The patient needs extensive investigation.
   D ESR is higher in men than women.
   E ESR is a useful screening test in asymptomatic elderly people.

Patient 90 Answers

| **1 E** Serum 25-OH Vitamin D. |

| **2 C** Multiple myeloma. |

This patient has hypercalcaemia, hyperphosphataemia, and renal impairment. Primary hyperparathyroidism and multiple myeloma are the most likely diagnoses. Both of these conditions can lead to renal impairment with secondary hyperphosphataemia. A parathyroid hormone assay, urine for Bence Jones proteins, and plasma protein electrophoresis are particularly important. Sarcoidosis can lead to hypercalcaemia and renal impairment although this is rare in old age. A chest radiograph is useful in exploring this possibility. This woman is likely to have a low serum vitamin D level. In addition, hypercalcaemia due to vitamin D toxicity is usually mild and would not explain this presentation, therefore measuring the blood vitamin D level is the least useful investigation.

The radiograph shows punched out lesions in the right hip (**90b**, arrows). The patient's presentation and radiological findings are highly indicative of the diagnosis.

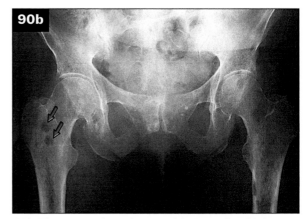

90b The arrows show the typical lesions of multiple myeloma.

Patient 91 Answer

| **1 A** ESR rises with age. |

Though an ESR of 50 mm/h is above the most commonly quoted normal range (<30 mm/h) for a women of this age, it is not unusual in very aged people to have an ESR at this level and to have no illness and no abnormalities found on investigation. As she is otherwise asymptomatic there is no need for extensive investigation.

Tutorial

The ESR is an indirect measure of acute phase plasma proteins, particularly fibrinogen. Fibrinogen is known to increase with age and consequently the ESR tends to increase with age. There is no agreement as to the normal range for increasing age. Accepted normal ranges now span from 0–35 mm/h for older men and 0–53 mm/h for older women. Its value in the range of 30–70 mm/h is therefore limited in old age because it is nonspecific and not always an accurate marker of disease processes. However, it can be useful in patients who are nonspecifically unwell. An ESR of more than a 100 mm/h should always ring alarm bells and lead to active investigation to exclude a number of conditions that can cause a high ESR, as highlighted in *Table 91*.

Table 91 *Conditions causing a very high ESR*
- TB
- Temporal arteritis (polymyalgia rheumatica)
- RA
- Multiple myeloma
- Blood dyscrasias
- Malignancies (e.g. cancer head of pancreas)
- Renal disease
- Connective tissue disease
- Occult infection (e.g. pelvic abscess)

Patient 92

An 87-year-old woman presented to the Outpatient Department complaining of tiredness. She had a medical history of DVT, MI, and a CVA.

1 Which of these statements is *least appropriate*?
   A The patient is polycythaemic.
   B She has a lymphoproliferative disease.
   C There is probable iron deficiency.
   D There is a thrombocytosis.
   E Patient could benefit from cytoreductive therapy.

Investigations (normal range)

Haemoglobin 13.2 g/dL (11.5–16.5)
Red blood cells 5.87 × 10^{12}/L (3.5–5.0)
Haematocrit 0.43 (0.36–0.47)
MCV 73 fL (80–96)
MCH 22 pg (28–32)
Total white cell count 11.4 × 10^9/L (4–11)
Neutrophil count 7.9 × 10^9/L (1.5–7.0)
Platelets 730 × 10^9/L (150–400)

Patient 93

An 84-year-old man presented to his GP with gradual loss of vision over 2 years.

1 Which of the following is the commonest cause of blindness in people aged 75 years and over?
   A Open angle glaucoma.
   B Closed angle glaucoma.
   C Retinitis pigmentosa.
   D Macular degeneration.
   E Cataracts.

Patient 94

An 80-year-old patient presented after an accidental fall. He said that he kept bumping into things that he could not see. His left fundus is shown (**94**).

1 What field defect is typically associated with the condition shown in Figure **94**?
   A Homonymous hemianopia.
   B Tunnel vision.
   C Bitemporal hemianopia.
   D Central scotoma.
   E No visual field loss.

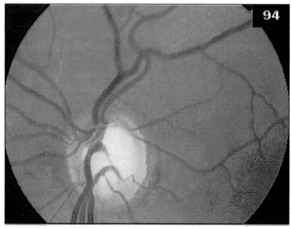

94 Photograph of the optic fundus.

Patient 92 Answer

1 B She has a lymphoproliferative disease.

This patient has an underlying myeloproliferative disorder. The indices indicate an iron deficient polycythaemia in that there is microcytosis and hypochromia with a raised RBC count. In addition, there is thrombocytosis. In view of her significant medical history of a DVT, MI, and CVA she should be given cytoreductive therapy to reduce her platelet count.

Patient 93 Answer

1 D Macular degeneration.

The prevalence of blindness, to World Health Organization criteria, ranges from 0.1% in subjects aged 55–64 years, to 3.9% in subjects aged 85 years or older; the prevalence of visual impairment ranges from 0.1% to 11.8%. For persons younger than 75 years, myopic degeneration and optic neuropathy are the most important causes of impaired vision. For persons aged 75 years or older, age-related macular degeneration is the major cause of the increased prevalence of blindness, whereas age-related cataracts predominantly cause the increased prevalence of visual impairment.

Tutorial

AMD, also known as SMD, is a degenerative retinal disease affecting the macula of aged people. There are two types, 'dry' and 'wet'. The dry type is more common and is more benign. It occurs in about 90% of all AMD patients. Most are asymptomatic. Any associated drop in vision is usually slow and mild. The dry type can transform into the wet type that is the major cause of blindness. In the wet type there is choroidal neovascularization. These abnormal vessels leak and bleed easily. If untreated, blood and exudate accumulate over the macular region. This damages the photoreceptor cells and eventually causes irreversible visual loss. The dry type is usually asymptomatic. In the wet type, patients may experience distortion of objects, blurring of central vision, or a scotoma.

Age is the most important risk factor but other risk factors have been identified. These include cigarette smoking, diet with a high content of saturated fat and cholesterol, AMD in one eye, excessive sunlight exposure, and a family history. Recently a gene predisposing to AMD has been identified enabling early screening for those at risk. Main treatment options include laser photocoagulation, macular surgery, and photodynamic therapy. Not all patients are suitable for treatment and the earlier the condition is identified the better. Most patients simply are not candidates for treatment either because they come too late, or the macular lesion is too centrally located, or the risk of surgery is too high.

Patient 94 Answer

1 B Tunnel vision.

The fundus shows cupping of the optic disc. This is indicative of open angle glaucoma. The patient was bumping into objects as a result of a visual field loss. Typically there is tunnel vision. A homonymous hemianopia is found as a result of a stroke or other damage to visual fibres posterior to the optic chiasma. Bitemporal hemianopia is found when a pituitary tumour is pressing on the central portion of the chiasma, and a central scotoma is found in patients with macular degeneration.

Tutorial (Patient 94)

There are two main types of glaucoma, open angle glaucoma (chronic simple) and closed angle glaucoma. Open angle glaucoma is the commonest. It results when the trabecular meshwork becomes blocked over several years, leading to a gradual increase in intraocular pressure and worsening of vision. The increased pressure inside the eye is painless as well as slow. If untreated the optic nerve is gradually damaged. Increasing age, family history, and Afro-Caribbean origin are risk factors. There is initial loss of peripheral vision and eventually the field of vision is reduced, so that only a small area of central vision remains (tunnel vision) before sight is lost completely.

Closed angle glaucoma (also called acute glaucoma) is much less common. It arises due to complete blockage of the trabecular meshwork, and can result in permanent blindness if not treated urgently. Symptoms usually affect only one eye, which becomes red and extremely painful. This may be accompanied by a headache, blurred vision, and vomiting. Closed angle glaucoma needs immediate treatment in hospital to preserve vision.

There are two other uncommon types of glaucoma: secondary glaucoma, in which the rise in internal eye pressure is the result of another eye condition such as iritis, and congenital glaucoma due to a physical abnormality of the eye present at birth.

Patient 95

A 77-year-old woman was brought to the Accident and Emergency Department by police officers. She had been found walking in the street, singing, and trying to engage in detailed conversations with passers-by. All attempts to take a history were hampered by her constant flow of speech, interjections, sexually explicit comments about members of staff, and a tendency to turn all questions into puns or word associations. There were no obvious hallucinations taking place and her thought content was not paranoid. She was not disorientated in place or person but had lost track of time. A call to her GP revealed no record of a previous illness of this type, though she had a history of depression requiring ECT about 10 years earlier. Her GP had not seen her for the past 2 years and she was not known to be taking any medications. On examination she was afebrile, with a GCS of 15. It was not possible to perform the AMTS. Pulse was 90 bpm and regular, heart sounds normal, BP 140/90 mmHg, JVP normal. Her respiratory rate was 18 and examination of the chest was normal. There were no abnormalities in her abdomen or skeleto-muscular system. Other than her mental state, CNS examination, though technically difficult to perform, revealed no obvious focal or lateralizing abnormalities. Her pupillary reactions were normal and her oxygen saturation on room air was 99%. Basic investigations including full blood count, renal function, electrolytes, screening liver function, thyroid function, blood glucose, ECG, and chest radiograph were all normal or satisfactory.

1 The most likely explanation for her presentation is:
A Amphetamine intoxication.
B Schizophrenia.
C Hypomania.
D Alcohol intoxication.
E Toxic confusional state.

2 What are the immediate dangers for the patient?

3 What short-term treatment measures might be needed at the time of presentation or shortly after?

4 Which of the following is likely to be the best for long-term control of the patient's mental state?
A Psychotherapy.
B SSRI.
C Benzodiazepine tranquillizer.
D Lithium.
E Psychoanalysis.

Patient 95 Answers

| 1 C Hypomania. | 4 D Lithium. |

The clinical features in this patient suggest that this is an episode of hypomania. The previous history of depression severe enough to require ECT is also supportive of that diagnosis. Amphetamine intoxication can cause a similar clinical picture, though it would be very unusual in an older person. If necessary, screening toxicology can be performed to detect amphetamine derivatives in the urine. The clinical picture is not really that of schizophrenia; acute onset of schizophrenia is relatively uncommon in older people and tends to have paranoid features. This patient has pressure of speech, sexual disinhibition, and an inappropriately humorous affect, all of which point towards hypomania, rather than an acute schizophrenia. Alcohol intoxication would normally lead to drowsiness and postural instability in an older patient, though there may be some disinhibition and aggression. Furthermore, alcohol can normally be detected on a patient's breath in such circumstances. In toxic confusional states disorientation dominates the clinical picture, and it is not usual for patients to have features of mood elevation, enhanced energy, and fluent speech. Nevertheless, both amphetamine intoxication and a toxic confusional state must remain in the differential diagnosis until all information has been properly assessed.

2 Patients with hypomania (and even more so if they have overt mania) can be a danger to themselves if they become exhausted through constant physical activity, lack of sleep, and risk taking. Some patients can also be a danger to others if they become aggressive or use objects carelessly and inappropriately. This can lead to a state of collapse in a patient of any age, but is more likely to occur in an older patient in whom physiological reserves are diminished by age-related changes and accumulated pathology. Patients with an uncontrolled hypomanic state can also become dehydrated and will also lose weight rapidly if they stop eating.

3 The management of hypomania, and bipolar affective disorders in general, requires the assistance of a psychiatrist. However, a clinician involved in the initial management of such a patient might need to start medications to control the features of the illness temporarily while waiting for psychiatric assessment. Atypical antipsychotic agents such as olanzapine and quetiapine have been found to be particularly useful for older patients with hypomania, though the older antipsychotic agents are also effective. Valproate is also a useful drug for bringing the acute features under rapid control to enable the patient to be more settled, sleep, eat, and drink. Attention also needs to be given to any immediate associated problems such as injuries and cardiac arrhythmias.

It is generally recommended that older patients presenting with hypomania should be offered treatment with long-term mood stabilizing medications, even if they have only had one episode of hypomania. The most tried and tested long-term mood stabilizing treatment is with lithium, though it has a narrow therapeutic index and requires monitoring. Of the drugs listed, lithium would therefore be the most appropriate. A more recently developed mood stabilizing drug, divalproex, is as effective as lithium or can be used in combination with lithium. It also has the benefit of requiring less monitoring. Some patients also require long-term treatment with neuroleptic agents, and it is usual to choose the atypical agents such as clozapine or olanzapine in difficult refractory bipolar disorders. It must be emphasized that there is a paucity of large clinical trial evidence comparing different treatment options for bipolar affective disorders in old age.

Tutorial

Although bipolar disorders are relatively uncommon in old age, they are important because of their severity and treatability. Most patients presenting with hypomania have a long history of depression with or without previous episodes of hypomania. However, there does appear to be a subgroup of patients who tend to present in older age and in whom there is either no previous record of depression or a long latent period after depression in middle age. The patient described above falls into that category and the lack of historical context makes the diagnosis more difficult in such circumstances. Although some studies have suggested that older patients presenting with hypomania have background cognitive impairment, it has to be emphasized that hypomania is not usually a manifestation of established dementias. Furthermore, there does appear to be some association between late-onset mania and cerebrovascular disease, particularly in patients with evidence of vascular damage in the temporal or frontal regions.

Another risk factor is head trauma, though the mechanism is not known. Other important risk factors are a family history of mood disorders and vascular risk factors such as hypertension and diabetes mellitus. Patients with late-onset mania should be investigated for underlying neurological disorders. However, it is not known whether control of risk factors has any long-term effect on the control of the affective disorder or the frequency and severity of recurrences.

Patient 96

An 85-year-old woman was admitted urgently to hospital with an acute confusional state. Her sister, with whom she lived, described the patient having several attacks of uncontrollable shivering the previous day. The GP had treated the patient for four episodes of culture-positive (*Escherichia coli*) UTI in the past 2 months. Her previous medical history included an appendicectomy 45 years earlier, hypertension, a benign breast lump, and primary hyperparathyroidism. Her current medication was amlodipine 5 mg daily. On examination her tympanic membrane temperature was 38.4°C, pulse 96 bpm and regular, heart sounds normal, BP 145/85 mmHg with no signs of cardiac failure. Examination of the chest was normal. CNS examination was normal except for the confusional state. There was tenderness in the suprapubic region on examination of the abdomen but no other abnormalities and, in particular, no flank tenderness. Skeleto-muscular system examination was normal apart from some mild osteoarthrotic changes.

The chest radiograph was reported as normal. Blood cultures grew *E.coli* in all bottles. After antibiotics and fluid replacement, the patient was greatly improved and no longer confused. At this stage an ultrasound of the abdomen was attempted but the views were poor because of severe constipation and inability of the patient to maintain a full bladder. A cystoscopy was performed which showed no abnormalities. Therefore, an IVU was arranged, a late film from which is shown (**96**).

---

1 What does the IVU show?

---

2 The underlying pathology is most likely to be:
  A Bladder tumour.
  B Ureteric stone.
  C Constipation.
  D Retroperitoneal fibrosis.
  E Congenital abnormality.

Investigations (normal range)

Haemoglobin 12.7 g/dL (11.5–16.5)
Total white cell count 18.4 × 10⁹/L (4–11)
Neutrophil count 16.1 × 10⁹/L (1.5–7)
ESR 40 mm/h (<30)
Serum urea 7.1 mmol/L (2.5–7.5)
Serum creatinine 90 µmol/L (60–110)
Serum sodium 138 mmol/L (137–144)
Serum potassium 4.0 mmol/L (3.5–4.9)
Serum corrected calcium 2.8 mmol/L (2.2–2.6)
Serum albumin 39 g/L (37–49)
Serum ALT 31 U/L (5–35)
Serum alkaline phosphatase 64 U/L (45–105)
Random blood glucose 4.5 mmol/L

96 IVU.

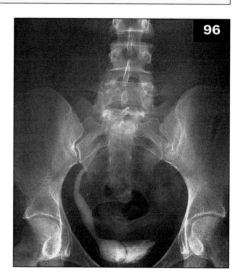

---

3 What might explain the recurrent UTIs?

---

4 How should this be treated?

Patient 97

A 75-year-old man presented to clinic complaining of a tremor of the outstretched hands. It had been getting gradually worse for about 12 years. He was increasingly prone to spilling cups of tea when trying to drink.

1 Which of the following statements is *least appropriate*:
  A The tremor might respond to propranolol.
  B Frequently such tremors are benign and familial.
  C The tremor is characteristic of Parkinson's disease.
  D It is likely to be worsened by anxiety.
  E It is likely to be improved by primidone.

Patient 96 Answers

1 The IVU (taken after the patient was treated for constipation) shows dilatation of the collecting system from the renal calyces down to the vesico-ureteric junction. The middle part of the right ureter is not visualized, though the lower third clearly shows a mild to moderate hydroureter. As this is a late film, the left kidney shows only a little residual contrast medium in the collecting system. This indicates there is some delay in excretion on the right as a result of the obstruction. However, both kidneys are excreting.

> 2 B Ureteric stone.

In this patient the most likely underlying pathology is a ureteric stone. This is suggested by the fact that the obstruction is at the vesico-ureteric junction (one of the sites at which a ureteric stone can become impacted) and the patient has two predisposing conditions for the formation of stones, namely hyperparathyroidism (which can predispose to the formation of stones caused by calcium salts) and hyperuricaemia (which can predispose to the formation of urate stones). A bladder tumour has been effectively ruled out by the normal cystoscopy. Constipation would not normally be expected to cause hydroureter, though it can, of course, cause retention of urine due to compressive obstruction of the urethra. Retroperitoneal fibrosis is uncommon and is usually associated with bilateral hydroureter. A congenital abnormality is more likely to have presented earlier in life and at this stage the right kidney would be expected to be nonfunctioning.

3 The presence of hydroureter can act as a reservoir for bacterial infection. Therefore, it is possible that this patient had recurrent *E.coli* UTIs due to persistent colonization by *E.coli* in the dilated right ureter. The fact that *E.coli* was grown on each occasion supports that contention. The prescription of antibiotics would merely clear the lower urinary tract but the presence of a reservoir of urine could result in incomplete eradication of the organism.

4 The patient should be treated acutely with antibiotics. Urological advice should be sought in patients such as this. It is likely that one of two options would be suggested. If a stone is still present, it might be possible to remove it via the per urethral route or by lithotripsy. If a stricture has formed, the lower ureter can sometimes be successfully stented. Re-establishing normal flow in the ureter will allow the hydroureter to settle, and should improve the function of the hydronephrotic kidney if performed in time. If the recurrent infection was due to persisting bacterial contamination, there is a high probability that this will not recur. Patients who are not suitable for such surgical treatments can sometimes be helped by giving long-term prophylactic antibiotics rotationally, though that approach is somewhat controversial and lacks a strong evidence base.

Patient 97 Answer

> 1 C The tremor is characteristic of Parkinson's disease.

In Parkinson's disease the tremor is usually seen at rest, though a mild action tremor might be seen. Action tremors are usually worsened by anxiety. An action tremor (sometimes called a benign essential tremor) can be familial and is rarely a consequence of serious neurological disease. It is easily distinguished from a cerebeller tremor by the lack of severe intention effect. Titubation of the head is an action tremor of the neck muscles. It is not a sign of Parkinson's disease and is usually benign. Propranolol is the first line choice for troublesome action tremors. If it is ineffective primidone in low doses may be effective. The tremor associated with Parkinson's disease can respond to L-dopa or dopamine agonists but usually the response to anticholinergic drugs is greater. Patients are best advised that tremor rarely disappears completely with treatment.

Patient 98

An 86-year-old ex-smoker presented complaining of headaches. He stopped smoking 3 years previously. He was noted to have odd shaped finger nails (**98a**). His funduscopic appearance is shown (**98b**).

1 What is the most likely diagnosis?
  A Cerebral abscess.
  B Benign intracranial hypertension.
  C Mesothelioma.
  D Metastatic cancer of the lung.
  E Primary cerebral tumour.

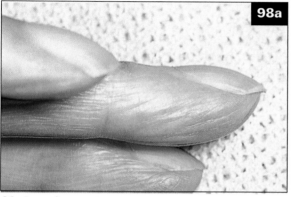

98a Lateral view of nails.

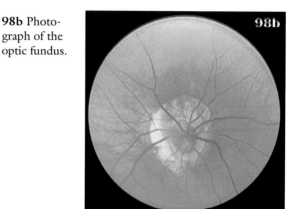

98b Photo-graph of the optic fundus.

Patient 99

A 75-year-old patient presented with a blackout that occurred while he was in the kitchen. There were no precipitating factors. A carotid sinus massage was performed. The tracing below was obtained (**99**). This was accompanied by symptoms of presyncope.

99 ECG tracing during carotid sinus massage.

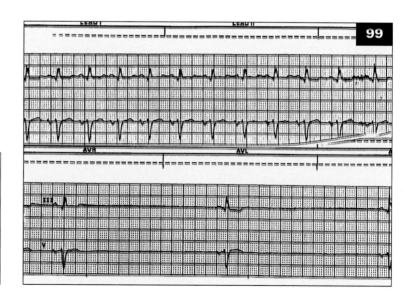

1 What term best describes the patient's condition?
  A Carotid sinus hypersensitivity.
  B Carotid sinus syndrome.
  C Vasodepressor syncope.
  D Complete heart block.
  E Situational syncope.

Patient 98 Answer

> **1 D** Metastatic cancer of the lung.

This patient has finger clubbing. His optic fundus shows papilloedema. The combination of signs together with a history of heavy smoking makes cancer of the lung with brain metastases the most likely diagnosis. The patient's left lateral chest radiograph below (**98c**) shows a mass suggestive of bronchogenic carcinoma (arrow), while the CT brain (**98d**) confirms multiple metastatic deposits (arrows).

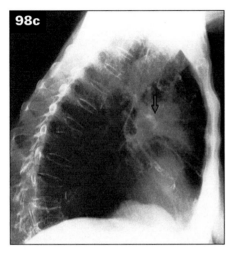

98c Left lateral chest radiograph showing a carcinoma of the lung.

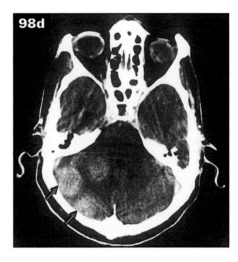

98d CT brain scan showing cerebral metastases.

Patient 99 Answer

> **1 B** Carotid sinus syndrome.

This patient has carotid sinus hypersensitivity. When patients with carotid sinus hypersensitivity have symptoms of syncope or presyncope they are said to have the carotid sinus syndrome. Patients with this condition can present with a ventricular pause of 3 seconds or more, or extreme bradycardia, as in this patient (cardio-inhibitory response). They may also present with a vasodepressor response, which refers to a drop of BP of 50 mmHg or more. Mixed responses also occur. Situational syncope refers to those forms of neurally-mediated syncope associated with specific scenarios, e.g. micturition, coughing, defecating, or arising from squatting. The mechanisms of hypotension differ in each case.

Tutorial

The prevalence of carotid sinus hypersensitivity increases with age. It is diagnosed by carotid sinus massage. This is performed by identifying the point of maximum carotid pulsation, usually at the level of the cricoid cartilage and rubbing longitudinally for 10 seconds. It is more usual to obtain a response on the right and the manoeuvre should be performed on the right first, followed after a short interval by the left side. It should be performed in the supine as well as standing position.

It is considered to be safe. However, there is approximately a 0.1% chance of permanent neurological damage and a 1% chance of transient neurological events. Patients should be warned and consent obtained before the procedure is performed. Rarely it may be associated with a prolonged period of asystole and resuscitation facilities should be available. Contraindications are the presence of a carotid bruit, a history of a TIA or a MI within the previous 3 months, or a previous history of ventricular fibrillation or ventricular tachycardia.

The presence of symptoms is crucial in making a diagnosis of carotid sinus syndrome because carotid sinus hypersensitivity may be present in asymptomatic elderly people. The condition is very effectively treated with the insertion of a dual chamber pacemaker when due to a cardioinhibitory response.

Patient 100

A 75-year-old woman presented with a stiff and painful right shoulder made worse by the recent onset of a rest tremor. Simple analgesia gave minimal relief. She was right-handed and was finding it difficult to write. She was also having difficulty with her ADL. There was no family history of tremor.

Further examination showed a mask-like face. She was bradykinetic and generally rigid. She had cogwheel rigidity in both arms. Reflexes were normal.

The patient was treated with Madopar 125 mg three times daily for 5 years. She then complained of periods of immobility alternating with involuntary movements of her face and upper limbs starting 2–3 hours after taking her medication. These were most distressing and did not allow the patient to sit still.

1 Which of the following is the most likely?
A Her symptoms may be due to a frozen shoulder.
B The presentation is typical of thyrotoxicosis.
C The tremor is suggestive of a cerebellar lesion.
D Polymyalgia rheumatica should be strongly suspected.
E She has benign essential tremor.

2 Which of the following is the best treatment option?
A Initial therapy with selegiline is indicated.
B L-dopa would produce a functional improvement.
C Treatment should be deferred to a later stage.
D The tremor would be best treated with a beta-blocker.
E Thalotomy is indicated.

3 Which of the following is the most likely?
A The patient has beginning-of-dose dyskinesia.
B Symptoms are due to L-dopa.
C The original diagnosis was incorrect.
D Treatment requires larger doses of L-dopa given more frequently.
E This is natural disease progression.

Patient 101

A 74-year-old woman with a history of hypertension, angina, and atrial fibrillation presented with general weakness and lethargy. Her BP was 160/85 mmHg. She was taking warfarin, isosorbide mononitrate, bendroflumethiazide, atenolol, and coproxamol. Her ECG is shown (**101a**).

1 On the basis of the ECG below which medication needs to be reviewed and stopped immediately?
A Warfarin.
B Isosorbide mononitrate.
C Bendroflumethiazide.
D Atenolol.
E Coproxamol.

101a ECG taken on initial assessment.

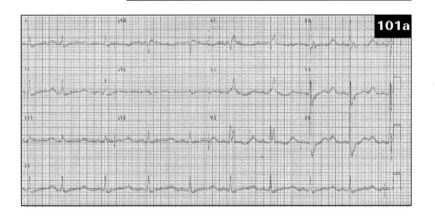

Patient 100 Answer

1 A Her symptoms may be due to a frozen shoulder.

This patient has a painful limb associated with a tremor. Benign essential tremor and a thyrotoxic tremor are almost always bilateral. A cerebellar tremor is an intention tremor ipsilateral to the lesion. Parkinson's disease is usually initially unilateral or asymmetrical and can result in a frozen shoulder that causes pain and stiffness.

2 B L-dopa would produce a functional improvement.

This woman has symptoms and signs of Parkinson's disease. She is having difficulty with carrying out her ADL so treatment needs to be started. It is generally accepted that it is best to delay treatment for Parkinson's until functional activity is impaired. Initial treatment is with a combination of levodopa and a peripheral decarboxylase inhibitor. This is most likely to improve the patient's symptoms and functional ability. In younger patients dopamine agonists are a better initial therapy. Selegiline is an adjunct to dopaminergic treatment but has little independent action. A contralateral thalotomy is reserved for patients with severe tremor unresponsive to medical treatment.

3 B Symptoms are due to L-dopa.

The patient has developed peak dose dyskinesia. Treatment is by reducing the dose of L-dopa and giving it more frequently. One must distinguish between beginning-of-dose dyskinesia, peak dose, and end-of-dose dyskinesia. Patients tolerate beginning-of-dose dyskinesia if given a larger dose of L-dopa less frequently. Dyskinesias are not the result of natural progression of Parkinson's disease but are a complication of long-term L-dopa treatment.

Tutorial

Idiopathic Parkinson's disease can be differentiated from other Parkinsonian syndromes using the UK Parkinson's Disease (UKPD) brain bank criteria (*Table 101*). This leads to a diagnostic accuracy of about 82%.

Table 101 *UKPD diagnostic criteria for Parkinson's disease*

- Bradykinesia (slowness and progressive decrease of amplitude of movement)
- Plus at least one of the following:
  - Resting tremor
  - Rigidity
  - Disordered posture, balance, and gait
- None of the following:
  - Recent neuroleptic, toxin, or drug exposure
  - Past history of encephalitis or oculogyric crisis
  - Stepwise stroke progression
  - Cerebellar or pyramidal signs
  - Severe autonomic failure
  - Supranuclear downward gaze paralysis
  - Cerebellar or frontal lobe tumours
  - Communicating hydrocephalus
- Clinical signs that may help to distinguish idiopathic Parkinson's disease from Parkinsonian disorders (multi system atrophy, progressive supranuclear palsy and dementia with Lewy bodies) are:
- Asymmetric onset of parkinsonism
- Good response to L-dopa and development of dyskinesias
- Absent pyramidal and occulomotor symptoms
- Absence of early memory disturbances (<2 years), hallucinations, confusional episodes unrelated to treatment
- Absence of early postural instability and falls

Patient 101 Answer

1 C Bendroflumethiazide.

The ECG shows sinus rhythm with first degree heart and block and right bundle branch block. The other prominent abnormality is the presence of U waves seen most prominently in V5 and V6. As the patient is in sinus rhythm the use of warfarin needs reviewing. However, the patient's past history of atrial fibrillation and possible paroxysmal atrial fibrillation need futher evaluation before stopping warfarin. The U waves suggest hypokalaemia and the diagnosis needs to be confirmed urgently. In fact, the serum potassium was 2.2 mmol/L. This is a recognized side-effect of bendroflumethiazide, so that drug needs to be stopped immediately. The serum potassium was corrected and the U waves disappeared as the ECG tracings below show (**101b, c**). Weakness and lethargy is associated with the use of all the other drugs. There is however, no other evidence of side-effects from their use in this patient and an alternative explanation needs to be found if symptoms persist after the potassium is corrected.

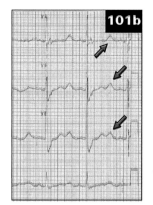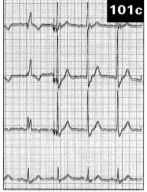

101b, c ECG changes during hypokalaemia and when the potassium level is normal.

Tutorial (Patient 101)

The other ECG features of hypokalaemia include prolongation of the PR interval and flattening of the T waves, as well as the prominent U waves. The finding of persistent U waves in the presence of a normal potassium should make a clinician consider the possiblity of hypomagnesaemia.

Patient 102

A 65-year-old patient with a history of advanced metastatic carcinoma of the bowel was admitted to hospital with a deterioration in his general condition. An ultrasound of the abdomen confirmed liver metastases. With nursing care his condition started improving again but 6 days postadmission he had a massive rectal bleed and was noted to be cold, clammy, and hypotensive. He was conscious and anxious.

1 What would be the most appropriate course of action?
   A Administer midazolam intravenously to control distress.
   B Administer diamorphine subcutaneously to control pain.
   C Administer diamorphine intravenously to control pain.
   D Administer fluids and group O blood.
   E Administer midazolam orally to control distress.

2 The patient died shortly after this event. What should happen next?
   A Inform the coroner.
   B Issue a death certificate.
   C Refer for a postmortem.
   D Request organ donation.
   E Sign a cremation form.

Patient 103

A patient with poor mobility due to RA attended clinic after having bought a Fischer walking stick. You were concerned that the stick was not appropriate for the patient and you proceeded to examine the stick.

1 Which of the following best describes the characteristics of walking sticks?
   A Fischer sticks are particularly useful in patients with arthritic hands because of moulded metal handles on which the hand rests comfortably.
   B The patient should grip the ferrule when holding the stick.
   C An angle of 25° of flexion at the elbow is desirable when holding the stick.
   D Patients with reduced visual acuity use sticks with alternating red and white stripes.
   E Quad sticks are not better than standard sticks at improving standing balance and gait performance in stroke patients.

Patient 102 Answers

> **1 A** Administer midazolam intravenously to control distress.

This patient has a terminal illness and the rectal bleed is a terminal event. In this scenario attempts to resuscitate the patient would not be justified as they are not likely to be successful or to lead to improvement in the patient's condition in the long run. Information from the patient taken beforehand in the form of an advance directive, or a conversation with the patient to ascertain his wishes can help this process. The content of such a conversation should be well documented. After implementation of the Mental Capacity Act in 2007 a patient can, while he or she still has capacity, appoint one or more persons with lasting power of attorney for health and welfare to make such decisions, though such people are bound by the law to act in the interests of the patient.

A massive terminal haemorrhage is a major bleed usually of arterial origin from a patient in whom active treatment is not appropriate or not possible and which will probably lead to the patient's death. The aim of treatment is to sedate and relieve patient distress in these last minutes or hours of life. Medication needs to be given intravenously for immediate effect. Haemorrhage is not painful and an analgesic effect is often not needed. The most appropriate answer is therefore intravenous midazolam. Patients taking long-term benzodiazepines are tolerant to their sedative effects and larger doses might be required.

> **2 B** Issue a death certificate.

There is no need to refer to the coroner or to request a postmortem examination as the cause of the haemorrhage is likely to be his bowel malignancy. Not all deceased people are cremated. This depends on patient choice, cultural influences, and religious belief. The patient is not suitable for organ donation. It is the statutory duty of a doctor attending the patient during his/her last illness to issue a death certificate. A death certificate must not be issued by a doctor who has not attended the deceased during the last illness. In cases of doubt the issue of death certification needs to be discussed with the coroner's office (the Procurator Fiscal's office in Scotland).

Tutorial

The coroner should be informed of deaths in the following circumstances:
- Unknown cause of death.
- Patients admitted dead or death occurring within 24 hours of admission.
- Deaths occurring within 24 hours of an operation or administration of an anaesthetic. (This applies at any time if the death is felt to be due to either of the above.)
- If the doctor attending the patient has not seen him/ her within 14 days of the death.
- Traumatic death (including alleged traumatic death).
- Deaths due to industrial diseases even if these are only contributory factors. Such diseases include asbestosis, farmers lung, pneumoconiosis.
- Deaths of patients receiving industrial injury pensions if the injury is related to the cause of death.
- Deaths not thought to be from natural causes.
- Suicide or suspected suicide.
- Deaths resulting from criminal action or suspicious circumstances.
- Deaths in hospital of patients under legal custody, for example, if a patient is held under the Mental Health Act.
- Possibility of self neglect or neglect by others.
- Hypothermia as the cause of death.
- Food poisoning.
- Death related to acute or chronic alcoholism or abuse of drugs.
- Death related to medical mishap particularly if relatives have criticized the hospital.

Patient 103 Answer

> **1 E** Quad sticks are not better than standard sticks at improving standing balance and gait performance in stroke patients.

There is no evidence that quad sticks provide improved postural stability. Fischer sticks are useful in patients with deformed or arthritic hands as the handle is made of moulded plastic (not metal) that provides better support to the hand. The moulded handle distributes the pressure more evenly on the hand making it more comfortable to grip. The ferrule is the tip that covers the lower end of the stick, so should obviously not be held by the patient. The desired angle is 15° of flexion at the elbow. A stick that is too short will cause the user to lean to one side. If it is too long it will push the shoulder up.

It is often believed that using long sticks in stroke patients reduces overuse of the unaffected side There is no evidence to suggest that this is so. Patients with reduced visual acuity use white sticks while patients who are blind and deaf use sticks with red and white stripes.

Patient 104

An 85-year-old woman presented at the Outpatient Clinic complaining of weight loss, palpitations, and tiredness. She had a long history of atrial tachycardia and was taking amiodarone 100 mg daily for the past 3 years with good resolution of symptoms. Thyroid function at the time she started the drug was normal. On initial examination her neck was noted to be abnormal (**104**).

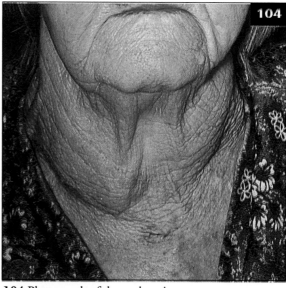

104 Photograph of the neck region.

Investigations (normal range)

Plasma free thyroxine 36 pmol/L (10–22)
TSH <0.01 mU/L (0.30–5.50)

---

1 What would be the best initial course of action?
  A Review thyroid function tests in 4 months.
  B Start carbimazole.
  C Stop amiodarone.
  D Partial thyroidectomy.
  E Radioactive iodine.

2 What does the abnormal neck suggest?
  A Multinodular goitre.
  B Grave's disease.
  C Amiodarone thyroiditis.
  D Thyroid carcinoma.
  E Thyroglossal cyst.

Patient 104 Answers

---

1 B Start carbimazole.

---

2 A Multinodular goitre.

This woman has symptoms of thyrotoxicosis together with thyroid function tests confirming the diagnosis. This requires treatment as soon as possible. Starting carbimazole is probably the best option. Stopping amiodarone would probably lead to a recurrence of the tachyarrhythmia and would not be the preferred choice. A partial thyroidectomy or radioiodine might be treatment modalities to be considered at a later stage.

The abnormal neck appearance is suggestive of a multinodular goitre. A thyroglossal cyst is usually found in the mid line. Thyroid carcinoma is diagnosed histologically and there are no features to suggest a malignant cause of the thyroid enlargement.

Tutorial

Amiodarone is commonly used for the treatment of cardiac arrhythmias. It has a high iodine content and a long half-life and commonly leads to disordered thyroid function. The urinary and plasma iodine levels are increased by as much as 40-fold. This high iodine load serves to block the uptake of iodine into the thyroid thereby reducing thyroid hormone synthesis (Wolff–Chaikoff effect). This effect usually lasts for 2 weeks and wears off. Failure of the gland to recover from this effect results in hypothyroidism. Amiodarone also blocks the conversion of thyroxine to T3. These changes often lead to a rise in the TSH.

Although abnormal thyroid function tests are common, intervention is not indicated if the patient is clinically euthyroid. Amiodarone can produce both hypothyroidism (commoner in iodine rich areas, e.g. UK, elderly, and female) and hyperthyroidism (commoner in iodine depleted areas, e.g. Italy and in males). Hypothyroidism is treated with thyroid replacement if the amiodarone cannot be safely discontinued. If the arrhythmia can be treated with another agent then the amiodarone can be replaced with a beta-blocker or flecainide. Patients usually become euthyroid after 2–4 weeks as the amiodarone has a prolonged washout period.

Two types of amiodarone-induced thyrotoxicosis are recognized. Type I occurs in patients with pre-existing thyroid pathology, e.g. a multinodular goitre. The high iodine load accelerates thyroid synthesis (Jed–Basedow effect). Inflammatory markers are normal. The aim of treatment is to block the synthesis of thyroid hormone by using carbimazole or propylthiouracil. Treatment is continued for 3–6 months in most cases. If the patient is euthyroid, radioablation is usually effective but in the presence of ongoing thyrotoxicosis it is ineffective and a subtotal or total thyroidectomy is indicated.

Type 2 results from amiodarone-mediated injury to thyroid tissue. The syndrome resembles a postviral thyroiditis. It is not always easy to distinguish between the two types. Inflammatory markers are raised. Carbimazole or propylthiouracil are ineffective and withdrawal of the amiodarone is best if this is possible. Prednisolone 30–60 mg can hasten recovery if the patient is symptomatic. Thyroidectomy is reserved for those not responding to medical treatment or if it is considered too risky to stop the amiodarone.

Patient 105

An 83-year-old woman was brought to the hospital by ambulance. She had been found on the floor of her kitchen by a neighbour. She was disorientated and drowsy; these were new clinical problems. There was no history of a similar illness. On examination her rectal temperature was 33.4°C, pulse 62 bpm, BP 130/80 mmHg, respiratory rate 10 per minute, and lung bases clear on auscultation. Abdominal examination showed mild tenderness in the left iliac fossa. CNS examination was normal except for a GCS score of 14/15. There were no obvious signs of trauma and her skin was intact. Twelve hours later, after spontaneous re-warming, her rectal temperature was 38.5°C, pulse 105 bpm and regular, BP 100/50 mmHg, respiratory rate 16 per minute. Her confusional state had worsened and the tenderness in the left iliac fossa persisted. With intravenous crystalloid fluids her urine output rose from 15 ml/h to 75 ml/h. Enquiries revealed that her GP had given her a course of amoxicillin 3 weeks earlier for suspected diverticulitis.

An ECG showed a sinus tachycardia but no other abnormality. Chest radiograph was reported as normal.

Investigations (normal range)

Haemoglobin 13.1 g/dL (11.5–16.5)
Total white cell count 23.1 × 10^9/L (4–11)
Neutrophil count 21.4 × 10^9/L (1.5–7)
ESR 41 mm/h (<30)
Urea 10.1 mmol/L (2.5–7.5)
Sodium 141 mmol/L (137–144)
Potassium 3.9 mmol/L (3.5–4.9)
Serum ALT 82 U/L (5–35)
Serum alkaline phosphatase 210 U/L (45–105)
Serum total bilirubin 39μ/L (1–22)
Serum albumin 42g/L (37–49)
Serum amylase 190 U/L (60–180)
Serum corrected calcium 2.3 mmol/L (2.2–2.6)
Serum phosphate 1.1 mmol/L (0.8–1.4)
Arterial PO_2 10.2kP (11.3–12.6) (breathing air)
Arterial PCO_2 4.6 kPa (4.7–6.0)
pH 7.36 (7.36–7.44)
Arterial blood bicarbonate 15 mmol/L (19–24)

1 Which of the following tests is most likely to yield clear diagnostic information?
A Echocardiogram.
B Ultrasound scan of the abdomen.
C Blood cultures.
D MSSU for culture.
E Sigmoidoscopy.

2 List the most likely diagnosis and the risk factors.

3 Which of the following is the most important next therapeutic step?
A Intravenous bicarbonate infusion.
B Intravenous cardiac dose dopamine.
C Intravenous antibiotics.
D Intravenous high volume colloid solution.
E Intravenous hydrocortisone.

4 During rewarming from severe hypothermia, the temperature range most commonly associated with severe cardiac arrhythmias is:
A 18–20°C.
B 24–26°C.
C 28–30°C.
D 32–34°C.
E 34–36°C.

Patient 105 Answers

1 C Blood cultures.

There is a number of features to indicate that the patient is in a septic state; these include the pyrexia evident after recovery from the hypothermia, hypotension, neutrophil leukocytosis, deranged liver function tests, and borderline acidosis. Therefore, blood cultures are most likely to yield firm diagnostic information. An echocardiogram might reveal reduced myocardial contractility in this patient if the myocardium is suppressed by sepsis or the acidosis. An ultrasound of the abdomen might reveal intra-abdominal masses or a fluid collection but would not identify the cause of sepsis. An MSSU, if negative, would help to rule out urinary tract infection but if positive (>100,000 bacteria and >10 leukocytes per high-powered field) could be misleading in an elderly patient since about 20% of patients at this age living in the community will have a positive MSSU. A sigmoidoscopy might help in resolving the cause of the left iliac fossa pain but would not provide specific information about the cause of the sepsis.

2 The most likely sequence of events in this case is that the patient has a source of infection, possibly diverticulitis in view of the history and the tenderness in the left iliac fossa, which has led to a septicaemic state. This is most likely to be a Gram-negative septicaemia in this context. It is probable that she collapsed because of her septicaemia and became hypothermic while on the floor in a cool environment. An alternative possibility is that she initially had a hypothermic response to septicaemia, which is a phenomenon that has been observed in some frail older patients, particularly with Gram-negative sepsis. The most likely mechanism in such cases is that Gram-negative endotoxins cause peripheral vasodilatation leading to rapid loss of body heat and a reduced BP. Although diverticular disease is the most likely risk factor in this patient, other important risk factors to be considered in patients presenting this way are recent instrumentation of the urinary tract or large bowel, urinary tract infection, and large bowel surgery (particularly if performed as an emergency). Patients in a frail, nutritionally depleted, or immunocompromised state are probably at higher risk.

3 C Intravenous antibiotics.

As there is good evidence of systemic sepsis in this patient, intravenous antibiotics should be given immediately. While awaiting blood cultures, an antibiotic regimen should be chosen to cover Gram-negative sepsis and anaerobic organisms, though clinicians should follow their local antibiotic policy when choosing the appropriate drugs. There is no need to use intravenous bicarbonate in this patient as the acidosis is marginal and would be expected to correct itself with control of the sepsis. The patient does not require cardiac dose dopamine because the hypotension is moderate and there are no other signs of cardiac failure. Furthermore, urine output has improved with intravenous crystalloid solutions, indicating well-preserved renal function. Similarly, there is no indication to give high volume colloids in this context; crystalloid solutions would probably suffice in this case, though some use of colloid solutions could be justified. The clinician needs to take care not to overload the patient to the point of precipitating pulmonary oedema. Some clinicians give intravenous hydrocortisone in these circumstances, though the evidence for its efficacy is not clear. Certainly, in this patient there was no evidence of adrenal insufficiency and she was not critically hypotensive.

4 D 32–34°C.

Observational studies have shown that severe, sometimes intractable and potentially fatal arrhythmias usually occur between the temperatures of 32 and 34°C during rewarming, with a peak incidence in one large study at 32.2°C. The myocardium is relatively stable at temperatures below 30°C and very stable in the 18–20°C range. Rewarming should take place at a rate of not greater than 1°C per hour if possible and the patient should not be physically disturbed while passing through the high-risk range. There is no clear-cut evidence of benefit in giving prophylactic antiarrhythmic drugs such as lignocaine, though that may be required therapeutically if an arrhythmia occurs.

Tutorial (Patient 105)

Patients presenting with hypothermia should always be investigated for predisposing conditions once they have returned to a normal body temperature. In some patients there is a clear-cut reversible cause as was the case in the patient described above. In others, there has been severe environmental exposure due, for example, to a fall outdoors in cold weather. Important predisposing factors include hypothyroidism, dementia (failure to take effective action in cold weather, and impaired thermoregulation), drugs with vasodilating properties, such as alpha-blockers and long-acting nitrates, any form of sedation that can blunt the patient's response to a cold environment, neuropathies that blunt the normal responses to cold (particularly in patients with mixed sensory and autonomic neuropathy in conditions such as diabetes mellitus), alcohol abuse, and environmental factors such as an inadequately heated house. This list is by no means exhaustive.

There is case observational evidence that patients who have presented with hypothermia without a clear-cut precipitating cause have intrinsically disordered thermoregulation, probably as a result of degenerative changes in the region of the hypothalamus. Such patients remain at risk of hypothermia and there is some evidence that they are also at risk of hyperpyrexia when the environmental conditions are hot.

Patient 106

An 80-year-old woman was found lying on the pavement outside her house by a passerby. She was difficult to rouse. An ambulance was summoned and she was taken to hospital. On arrival she was verbally abusive to staff, started to wander about, and had two falls. On examination there were knee abrasions in various stages of healing and numerous bruises, including a head injury. Her GCS was 13/15. She was afebrile. Examination of the cardiovascular system, chest, abdomen, and skin was otherwise unremarkable. Nervous system examination showed unsteadiness of gait with globally poor co-ordination and sustained nystagmus in both extremes of lateral gaze. There was no smell of alcohol on her breath. Her son said that his mother was a heavy drinker of gin and tonic (since being widowed 3 years earlier) but had recently had an attack of the flu and had not been able to go shopping for several days. He also mentioned that she had not been eating properly for the last year and had lost some weight.

Serum salicylates, alcohol, and paracetamol were not detected. Oxygen saturation was 98% on air. Routine urinalysis was negative. An urgent CT head scan showed mild atrophy.

1 In addition to general care, the most appropriate next step in her management is:
A Intravenous infusion of 5% dextrose.
B Intramuscular injection of 5 mg haloperidol.
C Nurse with cot sides on the bed.
D Intravenous infusion of B group vitamins.
E Low-dose subcutaneous morphine.

2 What other therapeutic measures are likely to be needed?

3 Discuss the likelihood of the patient being able to stop or moderate her drinking.

4 If the patient had a sustained convulsion on day 2 of the admission, the best choice of treatment would be:
A Intravenous diazepam.
B Intravenous fosphenytoin.
C Intravenous phenobarbitone.
D Rectal diazepam.
E Rectal paraldehyde.

Investigations (normal range)

Haemoglobin 11.2 g/dL (11.5–16)
MCV 104 fl (80–99)
Total white cell count 8.2×10^9/L (4-11)
ESR 25 mm/h (<30)
Serum sodium 137 mmol/L (137–144)
Serum potassium 4.4 mmol/L (3.5–4.9)
Serum urea 2.8 mmol/L (2.5–7.5)
Serum albumin 30 g/L (37–49)
Serum bilirubin 10 µmol/L (1–22)
Serum ALT 56 U/L (5–35)
Blood glucose (assumed fasting) 4.1 mmol/L (3–6)
Plasma free thyroxine 13 pmol/L (10–22)

Patient 106 Answers

1 D Intravenous infusion of B group vitamins.

The clinical picture suggests an early Wernicke's encephalopathy. This is supported by the fact that the patient is known to drink heavily, has been taking an inadequate diet, is not currently intoxicated, and has cerebellar dysfunction and a mild confusional state. There are no other features of an overt alcohol withdrawal syndrome, such as hallucinations, paranoia, tremor, or craving, so in the first instance it would be sensible to start by giving vitamin B supplements by intravenous injection (thiamine is the critically deficient nutrient in Wernicke's). Patients with thiamine deficiency are particularly vulnerable when they start to eat carbohydrates as this increases thiamine demand and can precipitate the neurological decompensation.

2 Despite the answer above, it must be kept in mind that such a patient could develop a florid alcohol withdrawal syndrome in which case it might be necessary to manage the withdrawal phase with a benzodiazepine such as chlordiazepoxide. These drugs attenuate the symptoms and reduce the incidence of convulsions. A reducing dosage regimen over 7–14 days is usually required. Clomethiazole is also effective but is restricted to inpatient use as it can cause dependence.

It is also important to investigate and manage any associated injuries, co-morbidities, and nutritional deficiencies during the initial phase of treatment. The INR should be measured and, if low, vitamin K should be given. There is evidence that sustained heavy alcohol consumption has compromised the patients health (weight loss, self-neglect, high MCV, high ALT, low urea), so careful attention to the nutritional issues is important, and might require the advice of a dietician.

3 The patient's alcohol abuse appears to have a relatively short history and was probably precipitated by the loss of her husband. In such a person there might be a treatable underlying depression or an isolated social state that could be ameliorated, in which case she might be able to reduce or stop drinking. In patients with a long-term history of heavy drinking the chances of remaining sober are much less. Patients with physical illnesses are also less likely to be able to stop drinking. Once the patient has recovered from the immediate physical problems it is vital to take a serious view of the alcohol dependence and involve the appropriate agencies to manage the condition after discharge back to the community.

4 A Intravenous diazepam.

Any of the preparations listed would be effective, though if intravenous access is possible the drug of choice is intravenous diazepam. Diazepam is less likely to depress respiration than phenobarbitone, and usually has a more immediate effect than a fosphenytoin infusion (fosphenytoin is a prodrug of phenytoin). The rectal route is slower than intravenous, though is an effective alternative if venous access is difficult. Paraldehyde can cause rectal irritation, though it is effective and causes little respiratory depression. However, most clinicians are more familiar with the use of diazepam suppositories, which are easy to administer.

Patient 107

A 90-year-old man presented with a long history of shortness of breath. A chest radiograph taken on admission is shown (**107a**).

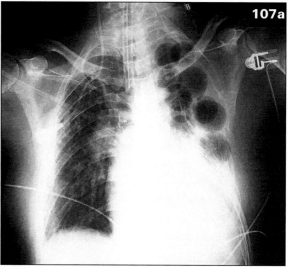

107a Chest radiograph taken on admission.

1 Which of the following terms best describes the radiological appearance?
   A Active TB.
   B Inactive TB.
   C Plombage.
   D Actinomycosis infection.
   E Thoracoplasty.

Patient 108

An 85-year-old man presented with a 5-year history of right arm pain. His upper arm radiograph is shown (**108**).

108 Radiograph of humerus.

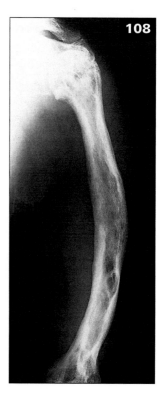

Investigations (normal range)

ESR 18 mm/h (<20)
Corrected serum calcium 2.5 mmol/L (2.2–2.6)
Serum phosphate 1.4 mmol/L (0.8–1.4)
Serum albumin 35 g/L (37–49),
Serum alkaline phosphatase 300 U/L (45–105)
Urinary calcium excretion 8.9 mmol/24 h
   (2.5–7.5)
Urinary hydroxyproline excretion raised

1 What is the most likely diagnosis?
   A Osteomalacia.
   B Osteomyelitis.
   C Paget's disease of bone.
   D Multiple myeloma.
   E OA.

Patient 107 Answer

1 C Plombage.

Although the film is rotated, there are multiple ring shadows of equal size at the apex of the left lung. The architecture of the left lung is distorted with collapse of the whole lung. There are no visible lung markings. This is the appearance of plombage. A plombage operation was used in patients with active TB to promote healing before the antibiotic era. For thoracoplasty ribs are resected to remove diseased lung tissue and/or to collapse a part of a lung. The appearance of the chest following a thoracoplasty is shown below (107b).

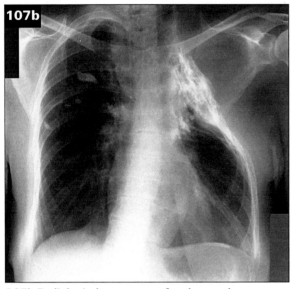

107b Radiological appearance after thoracoplasty.

Tutorial

Plombage was a form of treatment for TB whereby polystyrene spheres were inserted into the thoracic cavity to collapse the lung. It was a form of therapy used in the 1950s. In some countries it is occasionally still used to treat patients with multi drug-resistant mycobacteria at high risk of treatment failure and who are considered unsuitable for lung resection. There was no added technical advantage of doing a plombage operation over a thoracoplasty, other than for cosmetic reasons. The most common complication after plombage was dyspnoea due to the collection of fluid around the spheres and the loss of functioning lung. Infection often resulted in chronic discharging sinuses that were very difficult to treat.

Tutorial

There has been a recent resurgence of TB. This is not only accounted for by an increase in young immuno-suppressed patients but is also seen in elderly patients. Those living in poor conditions, such as the homeless, are particularly at risk. Those living in institutions are at risk as an index case can cause a major outbreak. Medications such as steroids can reactivate TB. It is, however, unclear how the ageing process and its associated impaired immune function increases risk. The Mantoux test involves the intradermal injection of tuberculin. A positive result is at least 5 mm of induration measured 48–96 hours later. Many elderly people are tuberculin-negative indicating decreased recent exposure; however, elderly people, particularly those who are malnourished or immunosuppressed, may also give a negative result even if there is active infection. In cases of high clinical suspicion but without microbiological evidence of TB, the clinical state may require treatment while results of culture are awaited. Attention should be given to nutrition as TB patients are almost invariably malnourished.

Patient 108 Answer

1 C Paget's disease of bone.

The most likely diagnosis is Paget's disease of bone. There may be secondary OA but this diagnosis would not cause the abnormal biochemical findings. The raised alkaline phosphatase indicates increased osteoblastic activity, while the increased urinary hydroxyproline reflects the increased osteoclastic activity found in Paget's disease of bone. In myeloma one would not expect to see a raised alkaline phosphatase. The radiological features with bowing of the bone and loss of the normal bony architecture also support the diagnosis.

Patient 109

An 82-year-old man was admitted as an emergency with a severe headache and inability to stand. He had vomited several times in the preceding 6 hours. All these symptoms had started suddenly while he was working in his garden. Until this illness he had been functioning well and was the main carer for his wife who suffered from Alzheimer's disease. He had a history of hypertension and had had a pacemaker inserted for complete heart block 3 years earlier. He was an ex-smoker. His medications consisted of diltiazem slow release 160 mg daily, bendroflumethiazide 2.5 mg daily, aspirin 75 mg daily, and bezafibrate modified release 400 mg daily. On examination he had a GCS score of 15/15 and was clearly *compos mentis*, though his speech was dysarthric. His AMTS was 8/10. His pulse was 70 bpm and regular, heart sounds normal, BP 160/85 mmHg, JVP normal. Examination of the chest and abdomen was entirely normal. CNS examination revealed incoordination with past-pointing of his right arm and he was unable to stand due to severe ataxia, particularly in the right leg. There was no nystagmus and cranial nerve examination was normal.

An ECG showed a paced rhythm but no other important abnormalities and his chest radiograph showed a pacemaker *in situ* but was otherwise reported as normal. A CT head scan is shown (**109a**). About 6 hours after his admission he complained of chest pain and a repeat ECG at that time is shown in Figure **109b**.

Investigations (normal range)

Haemoglobin 14.2 g/dL (13–18)
Total white cell count 5.3 × 10⁹/L (4–11)
Serum urea 8.1 mmol/L (2.5–7.5)
Serum creatinine 115 µmol/L (60–110)
Serum sodium 139 mmol/L (137–144)
Serum potassium 3.6 mmol/L (3.5–4.9)
Serum albumin 42 g/L (37–49)
Serum total bilirubin 9 µmol/L (1–22)
Serum ALT 48 U/L (5–35)
Serum alkaline phosphatase 53 U/L (45–105)
Plasma free thyroxine 2 pmol/L (10–22)

109a Non-contrast CT head scan taken on admission.

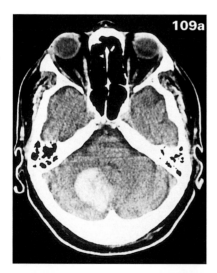

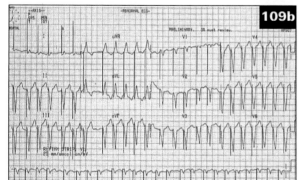

109b Repeat ECG taken during chest pain.

1 What does the CT head scan show?

2 The patient's main risk factor for this lesion is:
A Hyperlipidaemia.
B Paroxysmal tachycardia.
C Hypertension.
D Psychological stress.
E Smoking.

3 What does the ECG in Figure **109b** show? How should it be treated?

4 The most immediate drug therapy change should be:
A Thrombolysis.
B Add clopidogrel.
C Subcutaneous low-molecular weight heparin.
D Stop the aspirin.
E Stop the diltiazem.

5 What is the most likely reason for this patient's high ALT?

Patient 109 Answers

1 The CT head scan (109a) is at cerebellar level and shows a large radio-opaque lesion in the right cerebellar hemisphere close to the mid line. The appearance is typical of a cerebellar haemorrhage.

---

2 C Hypertension.

In this patient the most important risk factor for cerebellar or cerebral haemorrhage is hypertension. His smoking history contributes to the risk and it is likely, since he is taking bezafibrate, that a diagnosis of hyperlipidaemia has been made at some stage. However, there is no information as to the severity of that condition so it is not possible to contend that this is a major risk factor in this patient. Paroxysmal tachycardia can be a risk factor for thromboembolic stroke but is not seen as a significant risk factor for haemorrhagic stroke. There is no firm evidence that psychological stress is an independent risk factor for haemorrhagic strokes.

3 The ECG shows an irregular tachyarrhythmia with each complex preceded by a pacing spike. It is typical of the appearance of a so-called 'runaway' pacemaker. This is now an uncommon condition but has to be included in the differential diagnosis of a tachyarrhythmia in a patient

with a permanent pacemaker fitted. Some pacemakers can be reprogrammed externally, though if there is a fault that cannot be corrected, the pacemaker box will need to be changed.

---

4 D Stop the aspirin.

The patient is taking aspirin so this should be stopped. Any antiplatelet therapy can worsen a brain haemorrhage by allowing bleeding to extend. Thrombolysis will be contraindicated in this case and the addition of clopidogrel would simply worsen the tendency to bleeding. This would also be the case for low-molecular weight heparin. There would be no indication to stop the diltiazem unless the patient was hypotensive or had other adverse effects of that drug.

5 A slightly raised ALT level is a common and relatively nonspecific finding. It can be simply due to fatty infiltration of liver and is consequently a common finding in obese patients and heavy drinkers. Therefore, as this patient has truncal obesity, that is the most likely associated factor. Raised transaminase levels have also been reported in association with treatment with bezafibrate and diltiazem.

Index